Wellness Matters

Anthology Compiled and Co-Authored
by Dez Stephens

Co-Authored by Holistic Coaches
Trained by Radiant Health Institute

CONTENTS

Introduction

This anthology was created to inspire, motivate and engage you to figure out what "wellness matters" matter to you. Each chapter is based on what matters to various preeminent Holistic Coaches as they explore different areas of life such as passion, gardening, connection, music, love, ceremony, breath, pain and positivity.

This book is meant to be a smorgasbord of sorts. You can start at the beginning or really anywhere as the chapters are autonomous and each work well on their own – but especially as a collection. Think of it as cafeteria-style…you can walk down the line to pick and choose your daily dose of inspiration.

Many have come to realize that, "we teach what we need to learn." This bodes well for this collection of essays since many holistic coaches are seeking the same high standard of wellness that they encourage their clients to have and practice.

The thing to remember as your reading this book is that these particular subjects matter to these particular Holistic Coaches and may or may not matter to you. It is not meant to be a "how you should live" directive. We simply hope that this book ignites what matters to you and motivates you to allow that "wellness" to well up more in your life.

More information on these holistic coaches is available at RadiantCoaches.com.

Dez Stephens
founder, Radiant Health Institute

Wellness Matters

by Dez Stephens

Sometimes I wonder what my life would be like if I did everything well that matters to me. What if I completely took good care of myself at all times? What kind of life would I be living if I made a concerted effort to do all the things I've learned to be healthy and well?

For example, what if **physical** wellness was a priority for me? What if I got 10 hours of sleep each night to heal my body, balance my hormones, repair my cells, de-stress my psyche and completely rest my brain? How would I feel each morning when I awake to a rested body? Would it make a significant difference as I go through my day in terms of physical and mental energy? I'm guessing yes. I'm guessing I'd face the world each day with a clear head and a ready-to-go body. I'd have all the energy I need.

What about my **emotional** wellness? What if
spoke authentically at all times and expressed my
true feelings when it mattered most? What if, like a
child, I allowed my emotions to come into my
consciousness and then move through me
effortlessly? It would feel so good to just feel new
feelings and to not be constantly feeling old
feelings. I've noticed I hold on to ancient ones
sometimes.

What about my **social** life? What if I was more
proactive in socializing with others? What if I
spent time with people without having an agenda?
What if I didn't spend the majority of my social life
with my husband and sister? Maybe I'd learn and
grow in unimaginable ways. Maybe I'd talk less
and listen more...really listen...to everyone I meet
and get inspired by their stories and ideas. Maybe
I'd feel more alive inside because of all this new
energy.

What about my **financial** wellness? What if I let go

of financial fears and embraced a simple concept of abundance? What if I used positive affirmations throughout the day to reinforce my welcoming of financial freedom? "Money is everywhere. Money is my friend. There is more than enough money to go around for everyone. Money is easy to make. Money is available to me at any given time." Would this truly make a difference and reflect in my bank account balance? I know it can, because when I've tried these techniques before...and they've worked. So now it's time to ramp it up.

What about my **parenting**? What if I was simply more patient? When my 3-year old son is being obnoxious as 3-year olds are prone to be, what if I just let it roll off of me like a waterfall? What if I never raised my voice to him? What if I was more in the moment with him? What if I spent more time with my grown daughter instead of saying (in my mind) that we should do that more frequently? Maybe I'd be encouraged instead of discouraged. Parenting is not easy but maybe there's a way for me to make it easier. Parenting, by far, has been the biggest lesson-learning experience of my life. So maybe now it's time to learn these lessons with more grace.

What about my **spiritual** wellness? Now this is a tricky one. I've determined that I'm a spiritual person but not a religious person. But now what? I definitely feel spiritual in my everyday life but clearly there are ways to live more spiritually. Maybe I need to volunteer more to flex my humanitarian muscles. I know I need to meditate. Duh. What would change in my life if I did? What would be revealed to me if I did? What if I asked the universe to support me? Maybe more magic would show up.

What about the way I spend my **time**? What would unfold in my life if I could find the time to do the things I most love and stopped wasting time on less purposeful things? What would change about my daily routine if I decided to take control of where time comes from and how I expend it? Maybe I would never again say, "I don't have time for that." Maybe I would have all the time I need to do the things that need to get done plus all the things that I want to do. Maybe I would let go of the silly notion of having to do certain things I don't even like to do. Maybe my schedule would drastically change.

What about my **environment**? What if I drank the purest water and inhaled the purest air and ate the purest foods available to me? How would my life change if this became a priority? Maybe it would change what kind of shampoo and lotion I use. Maybe I would feel amazing. Maybe I would implement basic feng shui principles I've learned along the way. Maybe my home would flow better and open up more creativity.

Speaking of **creativity**, what about that? How would I express myself creatively if this became an important part of my life? What kinds of creative projects would develop? How might I feel differently if I was living a more creative life? Maybe I'd discover how creative I am. I might just surprise myself.

What if **played** more? How would I play? What kind of laughter would I experience if I was more playful? Would I play like a child or play as I am? Would I feel uncomfortable at first – probably. Would I get over it – probably. Would I have fun – you bet ya. Maybe I'd be the person others would say is so playful and fun to be around. Maybe I'd simply have more fun.

What about the wellness of my **community**? Would I become a more contributing factor to the prosperity of the people I live near? Would I become more plugged into the surrounding society in which I live? Maybe I'd contribute something important that made a difference for others. Maybe I'd become more interested in how I affect the world around me.

What about the wellness of the **planet**? Who would I be if I was more interested in positively changing the world? Would I focus on its cleanliness or maybe its human rights? Maybe I would volunteer outside my own community. Maybe I would donate to different causes. Maybe I would start acting on my heart's desire to help others. Maybe I would use the power of my intention to support everyone in every part of the world.

What about my **relationships**? What if I was more interested in fulfilling others instead of trying to get something from them? What if I was more generous? What if I stopped taking things so personally? Maybe I'd be less of a know-it-all. Maybe I'd stop judging people. Maybe I'd be open and honest. Maybe I'd be happier. Maybe I'd have healthier relationships. What a concept.

What about my **mental** wellness? What if I ate all the right "brain foods" and took supplements to produce a healthier mind? What if I did some of those mental exercises to increase my memory and function? Maybe I'd be more sharp and clear in my thinking. Maybe I'd retain more of what I want and release what I don't need. Maybe I'd be mentally void of stress.

What about my **sexual** wellness? What if I took Dr. Oz's advice and had sex at least twice per week? What kind of a difference would it make in my marriage, my health, my stress levels and my overall outlook? Maybe I'd get over some of my hang-ups about sex. Maybe I'd be more playful in the bedroom. Maybe I'd have healthy hormones racing through my veins.

What about my **intellectual** wellness? Would I read more to stimulate my cerebral self? Would I enjoy being a brainiac? Maybe I'd have more understanding about my world. Maybe I'd be more knowledgeable about how life works. Maybe I'd be more interesting in my conversations. Maybe not.

What about my **occupational** wellness? What if I took my passion and my boundless energy for my new business and focused on all the healthy parts of it? What kind of a business owner would I be if I set my intentions on a healthy bottom line, a healthy vision and a healthy implementation of my business goals and dreams? Maybe I'd have a profitable and thriving adventure. Maybe I'd be successful and prosperous beyond my wildest imagination.

I'm not trying to create a "perfect life" with all of these wellness components. I'm simply envisioning a life where wellness matters more to me than it ever has. So far, it has mattered to me mostly in theory. Now is the time for me to simply live well.

Believing in Myself Matters

by Kristianna Zack-Simmons

When I hear the words "believing in myself," I find myself instantly transported to a place that resembles a scene from a Disney movie. There I am dressed in rags with slumped shoulders, saddened eyes and a confused state of mind standing before a pink and blue fairy godmother-like being. She flitters and floats before me as I wait for her to deliver the profound magical words that will shift my consciousness and whole being in an instant. After the life-changing speech is delivered, she taps me on the head with her magic wand. I suddenly transform from a confused ragged girl into my authentic powerful self – fully aware of all my gifts and ready to utilize them. I hop into the black Mustang convertible she gifted me with and I drive off into the life of my dreams.

Why does this scene pop into my head when I hear

the words, "Believing in myself matters?"

It is because most of my life, I have not believed in myself. Most of my life has been with slumped shoulders, saddened eyes and a confused state of mind wishing for a fairy godmother to make everything better. I suppose I have had fairy godmothers in different forms. I have had friends, parents, boyfriends, students and my husband who all speak words to me like, "I believe in you. I will believe in you until you believe in yourself." They are always sweet and welcomed words but are not the magical words I imagine the pink and blue fairy would deliver to me.

I fully admit that not believing in myself has prevented me from living some of my dreams. For years I used to run around in circles chasing the same dream over and over again. I was fully supported in this dream. I had people believing in me. I had all my basic needs taken care of but I couldn't achieve anything or get ahead. I was scared. I was confused. I didn't realize it back then, but it was because I didn't believe in myself. I didn't believe I could become the person I dreamed of or change in the ways I wanted to. It wasn't until I started on a path of healing and recovery that I learned about self-esteem and "core issues." Not believing in myself was a core issue.

I have lived enough years now that I fully understand the only thing constant is change. Years ago when I started my self-healing journey, I was determined to give myself the chance to know what it would be like to live a life in which I believe in myself and know that I matter. I have been able to move forward and bring a few of my dreams into reality. I admit part of me still wishes for an actual fairy godmother to show up and bippity-boppity-boo me across the head and give me all the answers I seek. I know the answers that I seek are within me. I know the fairy godmother is inside of me. I know this because the magical words I imagined a fairy godmother would bestow upon me have come from my own healing journey. They help me navigate the changes that happen on my personal path. These words are powerful for they keep me in the now. They give me the power to shift my consciousness and allow the answers I seek to come from within. These words erase the projections of who I think I am and make me stand naked in the truth of who I really am.

The magical words are: "Do I BELIEVE in myself enough to make this commitment and go down this path?" and "Do I BELIEVE I can change?"

That is it.

When I ask these questions, I take my awareness within my body and wait for my answer. If my muscles tense and I feel restrictive, unsure and turn inward, then I know I have to do some work around strengthening my belief in myself. It may not even be a matter of believing in myself. It may be I am not meant to go down that path at all and my body is giving me the sign. If my body feels open, expansive, and certain, then I know I have a solid belief in myself to move forward. I know I am moving down the right path.

My personal healing path has led me to many discoveries about myself both profoundly beautiful and excruciatingly painful. It has taught me many lessons and I have acquired many tools for personal transformation and awareness. A couple of years ago, I decided to combine my personal experience and the tools that have served me. I created classes and workshops designed to bring people back to their "original self." I call this program Recovery Rising.

A workshop I teach from this program is called, "Roadblocks on Your Path to Change."

One of the first things I share in this workshop is, "Change can only happen and be successful if you

BELIEVE you can make the change." I remember the first time I taught this workshop and said those words. It was moving for me as the teacher because I was sharing a deep understanding and truth from my own experience. It was moving for the students because they had to get deeply honest with themselves. They were taking the time to go within and really ask, "Do I believe I can make this change?" What they were really asking was, "Do I believe in MYSELF enough to make this change?"

Asking those questions can save so much wasted time and energy. I do my best to not put myself down about the times I have tried to change my eating habits or venture down a new career path to only find myself beating myself up with words I would never say to my friend or family member because it didn't work out. I realized I did not succeed in shifting certain eating habits or flourishing at my new career venture because deep down I did not BELIEVE I could do it. I did not believe in myself enough to succeed. The truth was only revealed to me when I took the time to really use the magic words. "Do I believe in myself enough to make this commitment and go down this path?" "Do I believe I can change?" Now before I start anything new, I check in with these words.

I now stand at a new crossroads of change in my life. One road can take me into a new business venture and the other road can take me to lost dreams reawakened. Another road could possibly combine the two and create a new business adventure. The other road can keep me lost in a thick fog of uncertainty. I am not certain which road I will travel down, but I do know if I have to, I will dress up in a pink and blue fairy costume complete with wings and magic wand. I will look at myself in the mirror while tapping myself on the head and ask, "Do I believe in myself enough to make this commitment and go down this path?" I know these words will contain the magic that will keep me from going down the road of uncertainty. I know these words will help me stay authentic.

Yes. "Believing in Myself Matters!" It is truth. It is self-love. It is self-worth. Believing in myself is everything.

Now if I can just find some fairy dust to manifest that black Mustang convertible!

Breath Matters

by Ashiya Swan

Ancient Wisdom – Know Thyself

Carved on the back of a royal wooden chair found in the tomb of King Tutankhamen is the Pose of Immortality. This image of Shu, the Kemetic word for breath, displays honor for the ability to breathe and exist in physical form. Similar in status to the Lotus Position, the Pose of Immortality represents our potential for transformation when we are able to harness the surge of life force each breath holds. While the breath contains oxygen needed in our blood, the most important part of the breath is the presence of life force. In Kemetic Yoga, the purpose of this pose is to position the body to maximize the flow of this electro-magnetic energy up the spine and throughout the body. As we feel the flow of life force, restorative poses and deep meditation allow direct access to the energy of creation and the focus required to use it. From this understanding, what we now know as yoga was born.

Kemetic Yoga is the modern form of an ancient system of movement combined with breathing techniques to induce the flow of life force in the body for mental and physical well-being. The breath is used to flow from posture to posture, causing the body to become an extension of the breath. As we experience this flow, we extend the state of mind experienced during meditation to the yoga practice. When we create this meditative state while moving through yoga poses and postures, we create the ability to maintain the same balance as we move through our daily lives.

In ancient Egypt, yoga practice and breath flow was used for mental, physical and spiritual development. It was essential to prepare the individual for their life's purpose, chosen profession and ultimately, their contribution to their community. A committed yoga practice allows us to be healthy in mind, body and spirit which creates access to the Kemetic philosophy of Ma'at; the concept of universal harmony, balance and harmony. The time we spend in meditation opens us to the true reality of our nature. We are no longer entangled in the trials that keep us bound in worry and separate us from the peace and love of our true being. Meditative breathing allows us to experience the connection and solidarity to all that exists.

The Unity of Opposites

According to the science of yoga, creation occurs when forces that oppose each other find harmony and balance. In Kemetic philosophy, the concept of The Unity of Opposites maintains that two opposing forces should not try to dominate each other, but seek balance and harmony. To initiate and sustain healing in the body, we must balance the opposing aspects of the central nervous system, which can work against the body if we do not know how to respond to stressful circumstances. The autonomic nervous system is responsible for regulating our body in response to stress during the healing process. When we become stressed, the autonomic sympathetic nervous system responds by readying the body to protect itself against any perceived threat. Adrenaline and cortisol hormones are released slowing digestion to divert blood to the brain and other muscles; breathing, heart rate, and perspiration increase and muscles tense to prepare the body to fight or run. Additional sugars and fats are also released into the blood stream to provide fuel for muscles if needed. While we need our body to adapt to threats in our environment, unfortunately the body is unable to determine the source of stress or make adjustments to the intensity of the automatic response. The same process that occurs in response to a threat to our life or safety occurs when we meet the daily stresses of life. When we consider the amount of stress we meet in one day, we realize that our bodies are continually in fight or flight mode. As our bodies adjust to consistently elevated levels of these hormones that induce stress responses, we weaken our bodies and increase the risk of degenerative health disorders and harmful behaviors.

Breath matters because it can be used to initiate the internal mechanism for self-healing. Focused, controlled breathing is the tool used to physically counter the stress response. Conscious breathing initiates beneficial functions of the autonomic parasympathetic nervous system that cannot normally be controlled by the mind. Breathing ignites the parasympathetic nervous system, initiating the opposite stress responses and brings balance to the body through the release of endorphins, decreased heartbeat and blood pressure and improved blood flow to organs active in digestion. When the parasympathetic system is active, the brain emits alpha waves, allowing the body to move into a state of deep relaxation. We experience overall balance, calm and peace. This state of relaxation generates mental focus to we need to handle stress appropriately. As an added benefit, we gain increased clarity, self-control and discipline, which we can use to resolve the challenges and issues we face.

"If the Creator is everywhere then where are we? Are we not in the presence of God?"
– Yirser Ra Hotep

By acknowledging ourselves as holistic beings and recognizing the power of the breath of life, the separation we feel from the Creator becomes more apparent. However, when we engage in conscious breathing and meditative practice, we have the opportunity to shift our perspective. We no longer feel the need to connect to the Creator through meditation; we are reminded that we are always in the presence of the Creator. In this moment, we experience the power of our authentic self. Through committed breath work and meditation, we can heal the self-destructive behaviors that we engage in to try and fill that void. This meditative, relaxed state allows us to detach ourselves from anything that feeds the ego or the state of mind that causes us to feel that we are separate from the Creator.

The breath is the technology required to access our spirituality. As we focus on moving in concert with the breath in our yoga practice, we are able to unlock emotions that lay dormant in our spirit and block us from transcending our current circumstances. The movement of our yoga practice stirs any stagnant emotions and causes them to flow. As life evolves and we are faced with more choices and opportunity, we are also exposed to more stress and negative feedback from our environment. A dedicated meditation practice inspires the concentration and will power needed to use the energy we create to manifest our highest potential through meditation.

In meditation, we allow ourselves to release all inherited mindsets and conditioning we experience in life. We are also able to store energy within as a reserve for stress we may encounter during the day. If we are able to use this energy to rise above the ego mind, we can experience what Egyptologists call "Amenta" or heaven. In Ancient Egyptian thought, Amenta was not a physical place, but a state of mind that transcends any stress, negative thoughts or perceived limitations that block our spiritual growth. In order to access this state of mind we must use the breath to induce relaxation and concentration.

In the moment we are born, there is a pause of anticipation for our first breath. It did not matter if we expelled that breath with a whimper or a scream; it was simply delightful to hear the sound. It meant we were alive. In that breath of life, we became an extension of the Creator here on Earth. The breath is our primary source of energy used to nourish and bring the body to life. As we experience the stress of modern life, we can default to the involuntary nature of breathing and overlook the healing potential we have within. With time devoted to focused breathing exercises and meditation, we learn to nurture our divine connection and our potential as co-creators of our life.

As holistic healing becomes more dominant, the desire to experience life in a holistic manner becomes more apparent. Different modalities to heal the mind, body and spirit have separated us from ourselves. The impact of this separation is compounded by the fact that deep within, we feel the separation from our Creator. Modern science continues to validate ancient wisdom and we realize the depth that our breath matters. It is our connection to divine the source of life.

Ceremony Matters

by Lori Bradford Miles

The Practice of Ritual & Sacred
Ceremony for Creative Process

We change our consciousness, to create more
meditative energy in the world, to send out more
happiness, health, peace love and kindness.

A **ritual** is a set of actions, performed mainly for
symbolic value. A ritual may be performed on
specific occasions, or at the discretion of
individuals or communities. The purposes of
rituals are varied; with spiritual or emotional,
strengthening of social bonds, social and moral
education, or just for the pleasure of the ritual
itself.

A **ceremony** is an event of **ritual** significance,
performed on a special occasion.
Sacred - Holiness, or **sanctity**, is in general the

state of being **holy** as associated with the divine or **sacred**. It is what is considered worthy of spiritual respect or devotion; or inspiring awe or reverence among believers in a given set of spiritual ideas. In other contexts, "objects are often considered 'holy' or 'sacred' if used for spiritual purposes."

The practice of ritual and sacred ceremony as a creative process allows you to experience the sacred in everyday life through reflective living. Ritual is the form and structure that allows you to open to the deepest parts of your being. Ritual is the magic that you do for yourself which contributes to your wholeness by allowing you to access the sacred parts of yourself. A shift in consciousness starts to happens; a metamorphosis. Your entire life could be a profound ritual if lived with awareness and respect for ourselves, for all beings and all of creation. Conscious communion with sacred geometry is a fundamental aspect of our evolutionary awakening.

The truth is we are not separate and cannot continue to isolate from the environment in order to master, control and abuse it. Self-harming is the result because we are inseparable from the environment, and any abuse will turn back as a result of karma. The ego likes to control. In order to make progress in your evolution, the ego needs to be dissolved gradually, and consciousness expanded. What happens is the self-consciousness expanded, but also with this egotism. With attention primarily directed to the physical body and the physical world, one is hardly aware of the spiritual forces around him. Whether there is awareness or not, it does affect the spirit.

The soul seeks many, many experiences, often in the dark as well as the Light and as long as one engages in thinking, where one way is right and the other way is wrong, it is difficult to understand why the soul would make such a choice. But as the soul and as God are eternal in nature, all experiences are sought. It is the fabric of life, in a manner of speaking, to have infinite experiences, for an eternal soul has all the time in the world to experience anything and everything. With the aid of ritual, we learn to respect and nurture the natural environment. With awareness, sensitivity and patience, we can then learn to communicate with nature.

Take a walk in nature, in the mountains or in the desert. Take a deep breath and feel connected with what is around you. The natural cycle of all life, of all creation, is a succession of change and transformation. By tuning into these cycles through ritual we can attain a higher level of integration between ourselves and the world in which we live.

In ceremony, you are entering upon a journey of healing by transcending the limitations of duality. We call this greater power that we connect with – sacred ceremony to embrace life transitions.

Sacred ceremonies help us align our heart, mind, body and spirit, freeing us to live our heart's desires. Explore sacred places, special energy spots, crop circles and energy vortexes of the planet.

Sacred Geometry is a universal language that allows us to access ancient knowledge contained in our cellular memory. It is the key to understanding the nature and value of sound, light, love and creation. Primal Sound is the basis of all that exists, created and uncreated. As everything in nature and in the universe has its own sound, you can contact it all by its sound vibration.

Nature is a wonderful teacher. Listen to the sounds of its water flowing in a stream or a waterfall. Listen to the sounds and to the sounds within the sounds. Listen to and distinguish the different frequencies. Feel what these sounds do to your body, soul and spirit. Feel their vibration and rhythm, and sing, sing, sing. Sunlight makes life possible on this planet. You also receive light of the stars. When you enter the realms of Light you experience not only the living Light itself, but also it boundless love. The Light radiates an all-encompassing love and a wonderful, all-embracing acceptance. Light consciousness is a feeling of being filled with the Divine; with love, peace, joy and ecstasy. Love is a sacred surrender, to accept the fullness of life in all its expressions. It is this "love" that is the energy, fuel and movement that catalyses the energies from the confines of being human to that of being ecstatically and unconditionally in love with all of creation.

Sacred Geometry provides complete understanding and experience to consciously co-create a new world of Divine Expression and accelerate the Ascension process. In unforeseen forces, this encoded knowledge is information that is conveyed in signs and symbols all around the world.

The seeking of transcendence beyond the physical is being replaced with an embodying of that unified state of consciousness here, in every cell of our bodies. These new bodies are formed by the replication of new DNA codes. These dormant codes are awakened (to begin replicating) by light-filled sacred geometric shapes. The Language of Light as it flows from higher dimensions into our world holds an electromagnetic inscription encoded in the geometric shapes. The shapes of The point, The circle, The Sphere, Metatrons cube, Archimedean Solids, Perfect Right Triangles, Fractals and Recursive Geometries, Toroids, spirals, The Square Root of 3 and the Vesica Piscis, The Golden Ratio, The square root of 2, platonic solids are blueprint of Creation in all form. It is an ancient science that energy patterns create and unify all things and reveals the precise way that the energy of Creation organizes itself.

You will begin to see the wonderfully patterned

beauty of Creation. The molecules of our DNA, the cornea of our eye, snowflakes, pine cones, flower petals, diamond crystals, the branching of trees, a nautilus shell, the star we spin around, the galaxy we spiral within, the air we breathe, and all life forms as we know them emerge out of timeless geometric codes. These patterns and codes are symbolic of our own inner realm and the subtle structure of awareness. Golden Mean is the exact movement of creation in the expansion process. One is encountering and literally being BATHED in light "Golden Ratio."

Everyone will become conscious creators. Through this alchemical gateway, we bypass the analytical mind and connect directly with consciousness via the heart. This is where communication takes place with sincerity of heart. Your true identity will be revealed and the interconnectedness we naturally have with all of creation. It is a felt demonstration of how the power of the universe works.

What we experience is joy within the unification of our own existence. The sacred is everywhere, permeating in all of life. The sacred ceremony will continue to generate and continue to nourish the soul long after it is over. Ritual and ceremony are common features of this human life as there is a longing for connection with the magic and mystery of the cosmos.

Rituals offered our ancestors a glimpse of the divine order as well as a sense of belonging to something bigger. A new awareness is emerging in the world and many are turning to the rituals of the ancestors and ancients for help. They are working with ritual to unite families and communities to help them function with a healthy, balanced harmonious attitude to life and to bring a sense of spirituality into their lives in a meaningful expression of the sacred. They are looking to establish regular Sacred Place and Sacred Time. Here they can honor and support each other and allow spiritual expression to unfold, which will energize, rejuvenate and reconnect them with Nature and the Divine, bringing peace and joy to their hearts. Feel the core essence of Source, the source of all creation. Give your love and gratitude to Source for all that has been created in all the universes and all that has been created for you.

Begin with a silent meditation to allow access to tranquility and clarity. Set clear intentions and awareness with attention to the here and now. Notice not only what is happening at this very moment, but also the goodness, power and joy inherent in it. When you are completely present, you appreciate each moment one breath at a time. Acknowledge and affirm the oneness of ourselves, with each other and with the universe. Find gratitude, for it has the power to elevate you to an entirely new level of spirituality. Bring in humility as gratitude expands the heart. When you come from this place you can bear anything, transform anything and be the blessing you are destined to be in the world.

Create your own rituals with what you deem worthy. Though it may feel strange at first, creating rituals is powerful. When shared, you offer yourself, your creativity and your **guidance** in an activity that both grounds you in the here and now and invites a little magic into your life. You can create the container or the space. You can choose the space. Sacred Ceremony can be done in silence, reciting prayers, moving meditation such as yoga or walking, or just lighting candle to reflect.

Enjoy your Creative Nature!

My Own Personal Sacred Ceremony each day is to anoint the body. As far back as ancient times, bathing rituals are the key to total relaxation and to restoring equilibrium. This bath ritual, along with the therapeutic nature of water will nourish your skin and relax mind, body and soul. The therapeutic properties of water have remained a constant source of renewal or as a time of purification and cleansing. It's a chance to meditate and reflect upon the things you wish to wash away -- whether it's a bad habit, negative feelings or anything else. As you bathe, you literally rinse away what you choose to eliminate from your body, mind and spirit.

A bath ritual with lots of very warm water, nourishing oils, (almond, coconut, sesame) herbs, (rosemary, lavender) minerals, roots, tree bark, soaps, salts, flower pedals and candle light. All ingredients I use are organic and natural. I have created altars around my tub, in the widow sill above the tub and on top of a table. It is a letting go and relaxing into the space and allowing for gratitude to enter into the heart.

Try a ceremonious bath tonight.

Connection Matters

by Elizabeth Randles

The dictionary defines "connection" as: *the act or state of connecting, the state of being connected, anything that connects; association; relationship.* In our lives, we maintain many connections, in many different directions. Think of the web of connections running in your life right now and how this web affects you each and every day. If you had to prioritize your connections, who would be first? Your spouse? Your children? Your job? What is truly the most important connection in your life? What about your connection to yourself, to that soul part of you that is the Divine embodied? How connected are you to that part of who you are? Are you even aware of that part of yourself?

In our modern lives, we often focus so much on outer connections that this inner connection is somehow blurred, lost, and even forgotten. However, it is this inner self and our healthy connection to it that directly affects the health of our outer connections. For when we are connected to our own Divinity, to that own part of ourself that is God (or Goddess, or Source, etc.), we can connect to others and other things much more easily and healthily. When we come from a whole and healthy connection from within ourselves, we are able to connect more fully and freely with not only those around us, but with the world as a whole.

So, how do you know when you are connected to that God-self, that spirit within? We all know people who just seem to have this peacefulness to them, this self-assurance in who they are and what their place is in the universe. Oftentimes we compare ourselves and think that is what we must first achieve before we can connect with our true selves. However, quite the opposite is true. True connection with the Divinity of your own being is possible right this very minute, even if you are in the midst of chaos and disharmony in your life. This part of yourself is always there and always accessible, no matter who you are or what you are doing.

There are many ways to access this part of yourself, and it is as simpler than you might think. One of the easiest ways to connect with your divine self, your inner spirit, is as easy as getting outside and connecting with nature. There is a reason why we all feel more enlightened, more free and at peace when we are amongst the natural places of this planet. In connecting with and experiencing nature, we are brought back to our true selves – who we are as divine souls. Part of the reason for this is because being in nature, whether it is amongst the trees or near the ocean, is a cleansing and purifying experience. All the negative gunk we accumulate in our energy fields is wiped away, taken in by the earth and the air, and we return to modern life cleansed and refreshed. Even if you don't live near a forest or the ocean, you can gain the benefits of being out in nature simply by getting outside and putting your feet in the grass. By simply connecting our bare feet to the earth, we not only revitalize our systems, we also connect to the divinity of all that surrounds us. In connecting with the earth we are a part of the web of life that is part of every being on this planet. That, in and of itself, is connection to the divine, in both our individual selves and in the collective whole.

Another method of connecting with our divinity is through reconnecting with our inner child. There are many documented and practiced methods of connecting with our inner children, so if you feel drawn to one particular way of methodology of doing so, go for it! However, connecting with your inner child is as simple and as easy as allowing yourself to feel that childlike wonder and joy once again. One way to do this is to think back to your childhood and ask yourself what did you love to do as a child that you no longer do today? Did you spend hours playing on the playground or make up stories for your stuffed animals? Did you invite your "imaginary friends" to tea or run wild through the woods? All it takes to reconnect with that inner child is to find an activity you can do today that opens up that part of yourself once again. Maybe it isn't running through the woods, per se, but a stroll down the local greenway or even in your own neighborhood. Maybe it is as simple as taking a blanket, lying beneath the stars and finding the constellations. If you loved creative pursuits as a child, it could be as easy as buying a beginners watercolor set or taking a sculpture class to reopen that connection to your divine self. Allow yourself to feel, see, and be the way you did in your youth. Look at the world with young eyes and find that curious, joyful side of yourself that you still hold within. Above all, approach your new pursuits with the energy of a child – put aside your inner editor or critic that tells you how things "should" be or how you should do things and just do them. By allowing ourselves to connect with our inner children and do the things we love to do, we open up that pathway that is a direct link with the divinity within.

Another form of connection with the divine is in embracing our "shadow." Many people look at our shadow side as the bad or negative pieces of who we are. The shadow is the deep dark parts of our psyche that we often avoid and don't like to admit exist within us. The shadow side is the part of ourselves that may be narcissistic, controlling, addictive and manipulative. However, in order to connect with our own divinity and with who we truly are, we must embrace and accept our shadow aspects. How is embracing our negative traits or aspects connecting with our divine? When ignored, our shadow can wreak havoc on our lives. Have you ever found yourself acting out or behaving in a way you know isn't appropriate but you cannot stop yourself? Do you find yourself in certain situations and patterns over and over again? This is our shadow side coming out of the dark to let you know it is there. Instead of ignoring it and hoping it will go away, turning around, facing and embracing the "negative" aspects of who you are will make you more whole. In embracing our shadow aspects, and learning from situations that arise when it comes to the forefront, we connect more fully with who we really are. When you embrace your shadow self in addition to the rest of who you are, you will be more fully connected to the divinity within and more fully able to live your life in connection to all that is.

Once you are connected to who you are and are truly feeling that divinity within, you will begin to notice the connections you feel to those things that are outside of yourself. Once you reconnect with your own inner God-source, you will then be able to more fully see this in others. Connection with oneself is the most important connection you can have, and one that will never be severed no matter who or what comes and goes in your life. In connecting with ourselves fully and allowing the Divine within to flow, we will be much more open to true connection with others and with all that is around us. When this connection to ourselves is (seemingly) disconnected or disrupted, that is when we forget who we are and either form unhealthy attachments to others or things or when we withdraw and feel disconnected from everything.

In truth, we are never disconnected from our source of divinity; that is just an illusion. The only issue that has occurred is a perceived disconnection from ourselves, and this begins the spiral of disconnection with all other things. Once we reconnect with our divine and who we are, we find that life itself is a joy to behold and to drink in fully. In igniting this connection, we can more easily create miracles and live the lives that give us the greatest fulfillment and joy. All it takes is one simple step and one foot in front of the other to go on the journey of connection to ourselves and ultimately connection with all that is. If you are feeling disconnected, ask yourself, "What one thing can I do today for myself to reconnect with my divinity?" What small step can you take to reconnect with who you truly are? It does not take moving a mountain to start the process of reconnection. Sometimes just picking up the first pebble is all you need to get the energy in motion to reconnect with yourself. Once you pick up the first pebble, it will be that much easier to pick up the second, then the third, fourth, and so on. Pretty soon you will look back and realize that the mountain has moved and so have you.

Everything Matters

by Bliss Wood

Have you ever been sitting with a friend, trying to make a decision on anything – from where to go, which movie to watch, what to eat, what to wear...anything – and their comment to you was "Oh, it doesn't matter."? Does that statement sound familiar? Maybe you can remember saying it yourself? We've all said it at one point or another in our lives but have we taken the time to understand what that ready-made reply really means?

"It doesn't matter." Really? "It" doesn't matter?

I've contemplated the essence of this statement many times, turning it over and over and upside down, backwards and forwards, philosophizing to the point of exhaustion and I have come to the conclusion that not only does "it matter," but

EVERY thing matters...to someone at some point.

I realize that "everything" is a pretty broad topic and understanding how it ALL matters might seem a little overwhelming. Overwhelming that is, until we can find a correlation between ourselves and the world outside of ourselves. Once we can see our connection to life and feel our kinship to other beings, we begin to understand such phrases as, "I am my brother's keeper" and "paths are many, truth is one." In this respect, "everything matters" takes on a whole new understanding.

For example, does it matter that I sit up straight or slouch in my chair? Does it matter if my sister eats green beans or peas? And what about chocolate, does it matter if I eat dark chocolate or milk chocolate? What about you? Does it matter if you or your partner chooses the restaurant this time? Does it matter who pays the bill?

For me, the choice between slouching or sitting up

straight makes the difference in my posture and my long-term health. Because I am a health fanatic, the choice I make to sit up straight definitely matters. Sitting up straight now assumes that I will be enjoying strong healthy bones and a healthy back as I age. It may not mean as much to someone else but it matters to me. Healthy aging ensures I will not be a burden on someone else.

Eating green beans verses peas is a very big issue for my sister. Green beans are her favorite vegetable. She has disliked peas ever since she was a little girl, so I would say that it definitely matters to her, the choice between green beans or peas.

Let's consider chocolate. How could it possibly matter if I eat dark or milk chocolate as long as I am eating chocolate? Right? The fact is dark chocolate has healing properties called polyphenols with antioxidants that boost my immune system if eaten in moderation. On the other hand, milk chocolate is just another sugary "candy" and doesn't have much if any healing abilities. Because health is of great importance to me, my chocolate choice matters! Someone else might choose milk chocolate for its great creamy taste and that matters to them.

Now it's your turn. Does it matter who chooses the restaurant? I bet you're shaking your head, wondering why would it matter who picks where you will go out? "It's no big deal," you say. Perhaps, but it IS a big deal to the person who has a craving for gourmet pizza while everyone else in their group wants sushi. It could matter even more to the person who has a challenge making a decision and always defers to someone else, feeling like they never get what they want. We've all sat in the car and said "it doesn't matter" when our friend or spouse asked where we wanted to go for dinner and then we wished we would have been brave enough to request that little Italian bistro downtown with the red checkered table cloths, great cabernet and chocolate cannoli.

Think about how you felt when you deferred your choice to the other person. What happened? Did you secretly wish you could think of a better place to go than what your companion suggested? Did you feel relief that you didn't have to make a decision? Was your friend really happy they got to choose their favorite restaurant, and that in turn, made you feel good? One small choice affected everyone. It all mattered to someone.

All of these questions lead to my thought that everything matters, from the biggest decision you've ever made in your life to the most involuntary action of your beating heart. Each event evokes a level of consciousness in us. Even those off-color jokes or off-handed compliments that make you raise an eyebrow and ask yourself "what just happened" make a difference. They matter because they create change, no matter how large or small and change creates growth. With every thought, word or action, a reaction is established and thus, it creates change in everything. It is said that affecting one molecule can change the course of existence.

How can one tiny little molecule matter in the larger scheme of life? If you consider that everything is energy in varying degrees of density then you can see how we are all affected by this mysterious and powerful source that connects everyone. Everything, everywhere, at any time, matters to all of us. Huh?! In the words of our ancient teachers, we are all one.

Quantum physicists are just beginning to understand the correlations between thoughts, prayer, meditation, physical movement and manifestation. This is a concept that many spiritual seekers have known throughout the ages. Thoughts are things and they matter. What we say and how we say it matters. Taking action matters. Taking no action matters. Think about those times when you thought of your best friend and she called JUST as you were thinking of her. Did your thoughts about her cause her to call? Who can say for sure, but your thoughts and her call mattered.

How about that great advertising job you have, did it matter that you made the effort to apply for the ad specialist job instead of the mail clerk? Of course it did. Your focus on the specialist position, your education in that forum, your desire for the job and the connection you made with your interviewer all conspired for you to get the job. That matters not only to you, but also to the company you work for, your co-workers, your boss, family and friends. In short, it matters to everyone!

The point I'm trying to make is that there is a consequence in every thought, word and action we take and in that consequence lays a value and a reaction, no matter how small. The fact that something, anything has changed because of something we thought or did means that energy has adjusted itself to form matter which is a manifestation of that thought or action. In effect, something that matters to someone or something affects the whole universe.

To quote Albert Einstein's third law of motion, "For every action there is an equal and opposite reaction." In other words, if I offer to mow my neighbor's lawn because he is too busy at work, he may feel gratitude for my action which puts him in a better mood to deal with his stress. Because he feels less stressed for not having to mow the lawn, he in turn buys lunch for his assistant who is working overtime to help him. His assistant, appreciating her boss' kindness feels better about her job which makes her put more effort into her work. This also takes more stress off her boss (my neighbor). At this point, the assistant goes home to her family and is much more supportive and kind to them. They in turn, pass along the kindness they were given. When my neighbor comes home, he brings me dinner and I don't have to cook which saves me time and makes me feel good. Thus, I too

pass along my original act of kindness to my
neighbor.

As you can see, one action created a myriad of
reactions, all of which mattered to the people
involved. Forces result from interactions and those
interactions might be something as formless as a
thought or as forceful as nature's most ferocious
windstorm. Even Mother Nature acknowledges
that everything matters. She will create extreme
heat to create a spark in a dying forest and then
fan the flames with a gust of wind to start a fire,
which then burns the dead trees to the ground.
Everything is affected in that ecosystem by that
one little spark. That first wave of heat mattered to
everything in that charred forest. As well, that
same heat wave matters to the new life emerging
from the charred remains of the burnt timberland.

You see, there isn't one thought, one word, one
action that goes unnoticed by anything in this
energy field we call earth. Everything matters to

everything whether we consciously recognize it or not. So, the next time you catch yourself thinking "It doesn't matter," ask yourself what really matters to you. You just might find out...

Everything matters.

Gardening Matters

by Teri Pugh

Gardening: Cultivating or tending to the growth of.

Stay with me on this. As humans and individuals we are co-creators of our lives – our own garden if you will. What we focus on consciously or not, oftentimes manifests into our personal reality. This is not only true on the scale of our individual lives, but collectively can be true of our society, country – even our world. We make choices on a daily basis. Many are routine responses out of habit and lifestyle. Even as a result of our childhood belief system or circumstances, our choice in what we choose to believe becomes seeds which we sow in our personal garden. In the not so far-off future, they will become our circumstances. The by-product of sowing "weed seeds" is that soon what was designed and envisioned to be a loving, positive garden full of an abundant amount of happiness, compassion and awareness becomes overrun with judgment and cynical damaging thought patterns of ourselves and others.

In life, sometimes we get more hills than we do flatland but the good news is that a garden, so long as it's tended to, can flourish in any environment. It takes daily mindfulness to keep the positive in and the weeds out. Sometimes that can mean that we must not only shift or conscious thinking but also that we must consider setting boundaries for ourselves to ensure that we are the best gardener of our soul that we can be. Seems like a tall order doesn't it? Well, think of it this way...every word, every action, every thought we release into our immediate world sets in motion its own singular ripple effect. Don't fool yourself into thinking that what you say, what you do and what you feel do not have any effect on the world round you, most of all yourself.

Here's a simple example of a ripple effect. Say I hit the snooze button one too many times before getting up and getting ready for work. Once up, I'm rushing around the house, my dog Daisy is excited to see me and is wagging her tail and running around my feet and barking. Her growing affection annoys me as I am running late but in an attempt to avoid her I spill my coffee on my blouse and as a result, must change clothes. Now I'm further behind schedule. Daisy senses the anger in my voice as I command her to "go lay down" and she cowers away (I have chosen to respond in anger to the simplest act - Love). Moments later my child comes downstairs and is on Mommy repeat, "Mommy look, Mommy look" eager to show me her creative noodle necklace (if you're a parent it's likely you have at least one of these in your jewelry ensemble) but I'm beyond frustrated and frazzled, and out of an abrasive off the cuff re-action reply, "YES! I see…ANOTHER noodle necklace, it's not like I've not seen that before!" Feelings hurt, my daughter leaves the room (a kinder choice in words rather than split-second anger would have nurtured my child rather than planting a seed that "she" was the reason mommy was late or angry). Fast forward, in traffic, which I wouldn't have been had I not set in motion this chain of events by "choosing" to hit the snooze button one to many times. I notice a car trying desperately to edge over. Their turn signal on, patiently waiting they hope someone, okay - ME will be nice enough to let them cut in, but I'm already late and annoyed so I choose not let them over. What I didn't know was they were on their way to Hospice to see a dying family member. Feeling a false sense of victory having not let my fellow rush-hour neighbor over, I plow ahead. Soon I pull up upon a street vendor who is selling the local paper, rather than make eye contact and say "good morning" I choose to turn the other way, quickly rolling my window up to avoid making any contact with him at all, but he witnesses my hurried actions (a sense of defeat comes over him). Arriving at the office, I immediately run into a staff member, by now in full-blown "the world is against me mode," I lash out or worse, engage in a game of passive aggressive roulette. I chose to reply with a fairly sharp tongue which sets in motion yet another dangerous ripple effect.

Not only have I spread my negative weed seeds everywhere like a crop duster gone wild. I've now managed to toss them into others unsuspecting gardens. My dog, Daisy chews up my shoe that day. My daughter gets into trouble a preschool for screaming at another child. The man in traffic beats himself up for "not being there," the street vendor takes that forbidden drink. My co-worker goes home and unleashes his own fury on his wife and children as a result of our interactions earlier in the day. Are you seeing the trend here? We "choose." We choose to plant seeds of Love, Patience, Compassion and Kindness – or not too. Now this isn't to say that every day is cotton candy and ferris wheels by any means. After all, we're human and we expect that at some point we will have bad moments, but it's how we choose to "think" before we react, its how we choose to "think" before we speak that will determine how beautiful our garden grows. As humans, we somehow get consumed with the frantic pace of life unfolding around us and become desensitized by the ever-growing wave of detachment, cynicism and sadness that has slowly crept in on us. We've somehow forgotten the reality that we are part of a force greater than ourselves and we have a responsibility to spread kindness, compassion and love to those around us. As human beings we have the innate ability to change our behavior. Sometimes it's easy and sometimes it takes looking a bit deeper into the reason why we feel the way we do. And let's face it; there are some folks who would rather experience root canal before entertaining the notion that even for a second they might be part of the problem at hand. Still, this doesn't mean they can't dip their hand into that wheel barrel of kaka and pull out a delicate flower. Think about that the next time you are a one of those super centers buying your spring time starter bulbs. Each flower you see started off as a seed and their potential for becoming the best they could be was a direct result of a human tending to the garden.

If we find ourselves a bit off kilter as a result of too much negativity, perhaps it is time to readjust our thinking. If we have old wounds that simply refuse to heal, heartache, anger or grief that we have not yet processed and come to terms with, it's essential to our well-being and personal growth to address those issues. Having a new perspective on past pain can truly reshape your future. The simplest of mindful actions can set in motion ripple effects that can sweep our world, but no one can initiate that forward motion but us. When we truly desire to change our world, we will find that we gravitate toward that which supports us and enables us to reach our highest good. As we evolve, we continue to attract those positive people and circumstances that nurture us. This is

why gardening matters. Now go on; don't you have
some beautiful seeds to sow?

Music Matters

by Nancy Moran

It was summer, 1988. I was two years out of college and already a year into my second job, working for a small consulting firm in Rosslyn, Virginia. I was living the professional life and used to wearing suits, pantyhose and pumps. But on this particular afternoon, I was attending my office's summer barbecue at a local park. It was a casual and relaxed non-business affair. So, between my colleagues and all of our spouses, significant others, and children, there were about 20 of us in shorts and t-shirts, playing volleyball, eating hamburgers and drinking beer. At some point, the wife of my boss's boss started talking to me about the music group that I played in.

I had joined an acoustic band the year before as their female singer. We'd only done a few gigs together at some local bars and restaurants around town. But it was fun for me to sing with other musicians and I enjoyed covering songs like "Landslide" by Stevie Nicks and "Free Man in Paris" by Joni Mitchell. So, I was more than happy to talk to her about the group and music in general.

I don't really remember what I said to her. But I remember distinctly what she said to me. At the end of our conversation she said (in what I interpreted as a condescending tone), "Well, isn't that nice! Because someday you'll be able to look back on playing music and remember what a fun time it was."

I was shocked and stunned by her remark. And while I didn't say anything to her directly—she WAS the boss's boss wife after all—I remember feeling angry. How *dare* she assume that I won't be doing music later in life! How *dare* she imply that my music was a cute, little hobby that I would eventually grow out of when I grew up! Music was *way* more important than that!

And that was it.

THAT was the first moment I realized that *music matters*!

It would still take me a few years to realize that music was my calling and to leave the regular working-world behind. But that moment significantly changed me forever.

Now, you might be thinking, "Yeah, music is important to YOU because you're a musician and a singer."

And you might be right. Perhaps music matters more to me than it does to some people. I mean, I literally NEED the frequency vibrations of singing. It's part of what makes me, ME. I get an intangible benefit from singing that impacts my entire being and life. I feel complete when I play music...and I get a little cranky and out of sorts when I go too long without it.

But music isn't just for musicians and singers and songwriters. And I don't think it *matters* just because it's what I do for a living.

So how do I explain why and how music matters to people—not just to musicians, but to ALL people? How can I explain something that, in my mind, is so important, so vital, and so integral to our existence? It's a little like trying to explain why breathing matters. Or eating matters. Perhaps German philosopher Friedrich Nietzsche summed it up best when he wrote, "Without music, life would be a mistake."

Maybe I should start simply by defining it. What is music exactly? It's harmony and melody. It's rhythm and tempo and timing. It's tone and pitch and velocity and dynamics. It's frequency, notes and the spaces in between. Structure, beat and groove. It's passion, really. It's anger and sadness and love and joy. Heartbreak and hatred. Celebration and grieving. It's serious and playful, brooding and ominous, suspenseful and happy, bright and somber. It's ALL of these things in one; and none of them at the same time.

When you think about it, music is everywhere. Yes, it's in the obvious places like your car radio, home stereo, and iPod. But it's also on TV—in every show that you watch, every movie, and even most advertisements have music. It's being played in your grocery store, in shopping malls, and at your favorite restaurant. At the high school football game, there's a marching band. There's music at baseball games, football games, basketball games and hockey games. Motivational speakers use music to fire up an audience. Political candidates have musical themes to make a statement and/or unite their supporters. Most churches use music. There's even music when you're put on hold with your credit card customer service line. And heck!

What would a birthday party be without singing "Happy Birthday" to the guest of honor?

There's music to calm you down and to pump you up. Music to put you to sleep and to wake you up. Music to dance to, music to cry to, music to laugh with, and music to go back in time with. There's even music to help educate you. I mean, how did you learn your ABCs?

But is this why music *matters*?!?

Music doesn't matter simply because it exists. I believe music matters because it is a direct connection with spirit, heart, and soul. It's pure expression. It's intimate. Almost like sex.

Music expresses thoughts, ideas and feelings that can't be expressed with words alone. Ever had a word on the tip of your tongue and you can't quite find the right way to say EXACTLY what you mean? Music can express that. Music is the meaning that is implied. It's the read-between-the-lines. It is a deep, emotional language and a form of expression that comes from the innermost parts of our existence. And whether you believe you are musical or not, I believe it exists within you, the same way love, sadness, and anger exist within you. Music is integral to our being.

Because of this, music is highly individual; unique to each person. And thus, there are a wide variety of styles for each taste. Some people will be moved by the cellos in a symphony orchestra and others by the horn of Louis Armstrong. Some will call Rock and Roll noise while others just won't get the ramblings of jazz. Some will listen intently to the lyrics of a song, and some will hear the melody over anything else.

Music is also a way of connecting to PEOPLE— something I feel we desperately need in today's virtual environment. Whether you're listening to music alone in your car or with thousands of other people at a crowded stadium concert, music is meant to be *experienced*. And that experience connects you with other people—the songwriter, the musicians, the singer, and the other fans or audience members that also listen to and connect with the music.

Teenagers who dress in all black and listen to heavy metal are connecting with others who hear and feel the same thing in the music. Likewise, 50 year-olds who listen to folk music are connecting with others who "get" this type of music. That's not to say that you'll agree with everything in a particular style of music or that you'll like everyone who listens to the same type of music you listen to. But it does mean that you have something in common with other people on the planet. With music—even if you are playing it or listening to it by yourself—you are never alone.

Music transcends language, gender, race, age, ethnic and cultural boundaries. It helps us to understand and to be understood. It's a way to observe ourselves. It reflects and comments on society. It's all inclusive. It's inviting. And sometimes, it even breaks down barriers and walls between people.

Music matters because it can *change* people.

I once had an intuitive psychic tell me that I needed to sing more because using my voice to sing creates unique sound waves that no other person can produce. And she said the world needs my voice—my sound waves—to make the changes we need to make.

That's true for everyone. We need all forms of music—good music and bad; in tune and off key; professional and amateur; serious music and just goofing around ditties. Every bit of it is necessary in the scheme of our lives because it affects and changes us. That's the ripple effect to an extreme. And I personally believe it to be true. But it may sound woo-woo to some people—like my former boss's boss's wife—who think that music is just an accessory to life.

Looking back now, I probably should thank her. She certainly changed my mind about the importance of music and she just may be the reason that I'm doing music full time today! But you don't have to quit your day job or even play an instrument to enjoy and appreciate the power of music. You don't even have to attend a concert or buy a recording—although, as a professional musician, I highly suggest that you do. You can simply listen to the birds singing outside your bedroom window. Or to the wind as it rustles leaves or howls in between tall downtown buildings. Once you learn the language of music you will hear it all around you.

Many great things in life can't be explained. The Universe can't be explained. Love can't be explained. Music can't be explained.

And that's why it matters!

None of It Matters

by Jackie Almaguer

No, I'm not a Buddhist nun nor an existential philosopher. I'm Jackie – a woman with an appetite for life, love and art. I grew up all over the place, from the streets of Chicago to the wooded lands of Tennessee. In my short 30 years, I feel I'm a warrior – a survivor of life.

My parents were very young when they had me, my mother was 15 and my father was 18. They were merely children themselves with a baby on their hands. They were forced to marry and it only lasted a couple of years. My Mom moved to California, with me, when I was only two and to Tennessee when I was 17. I bounced between parents for the next 15 years and attended over seven different schools.

I don't like saying that I'm a victim of anything

because I'm still here. I prefer to say I'm a survivor. A survivor of sexual, physical, verbal and mental abuse and it all started when I was six. What happened to me then just created a domino affect for the rest of my life. One horrifying event after the next, and before I knew it I was drinking and doing heavy drugs just to numb the pain I called my life.

I felt alone and lost in a world with all the odds against me. It felt like I was so different from all the other girls and I wasn't good enough for any of the perks. I had many interests but didn't fit in anywhere. My religion didn't accept me because of my sexuality, family didn't appreciate me because I was the black sheep and society didn't want me because I was never able to conform to the norm.

I spiraled down real quick but I kept smiling and laughing so no one would even suspect how broken I was. I hated life and everyone in it. My relationship with my parents was so bad I felt like an orphan and I was constantly looking for older people to take that emotional place of my parents. Life just didn't seem worth living and I came real close to ending it.

But guess what? None of it Matters.

That's right, none of it matters because it happened in the past. It's now just a story, not History but MY-story. A story I chose to let run my life and determine who I could have been and what I was. A story that now only exists in my head. Although we all have wounds, and unless it has killed you, we also have the ability to heal regardless how deep that wound is. And since you are reading this, you can heal as well. Heal and move on; that's key to understanding that "None of it Matters."

As a society, we are taught to bury all secrets and never mend the open wounds. We are taught to cope with trauma but never nurse ourselves back to health. One of my favorite painters, Frida Kahlo, once said, "I drink to drown my sorrows, but the damn things learned to swim." That's what we do! Since we never deal with our sorrows (rape, violence, death, etc.), they keep resurfacing and showing up for us all of our life until the wound is healed. Instead we cover it up with alcohol, drugs, sex, food and self destruction to numb the pain.

Religion has taught us how to live in fear, hate those who are different and how NOT to love ourselves. Not everyone grew up in a religious setting so let me explain the Fear Factor. At a very young age, they teach you that if you don't do what God says (also what your parents say), He will come down for you and send you to Hell and burn for an eternity. Haven't you ever heard people say things like, "He's a God fearing man."? I went to a few Catholic schools and we had to confess every few days, all the "sins" we had committed. The constant reminder that we do bad things everyday puts fear into a child and molds the way they think for years to come. They also teach to hate those who are different and by different I don't mean handicapped or a midget. Different translates to everyone who doesn't believe what "they" believe or goes against their teachings. So if you are gay, bi-racial, Buddhist or anything else that doesn't conform to their religion, you are hated and not accepted. With all this hate and fear, how are we supposed to love one another and ourselves?

We don't! The hateful and fearing mindset causes us to hate ourselves because of the constant reminder that we are sinners and God will not love us, and how dare we love ourselves the way we are.

The media has taught us that we aren't perfect unless we look, talk, act, smell, feel and operate in a certain way. Things like magazines and TV shows that always tend to portray what a typical healthy woman or man should look like. Do you know what Photoshop is? Being a size two with blonde hair and perfect-size teeth doesn't mean healthy. Other media like the news focuses on every negative possible thing that could happen to humanity, from rape to murder and everything in between. I know it's good to stay informed of what happens around the world, but does it really empower you? With today's media, it is said that by the time a child reaches the age of 14, they would have witnesses over 10,000 deaths.

Our school system teaches children to regurgitate facts, become submissive to authority and remove all self-expression. It's like when the Native Americans were put into boarding schools. They were stripped of their culture and language and were taught to hate who they were as a People. That's what today's school system does. Take a look at the horrible processed food they serve, the uniforms they are forced to wear and the violence they experience during school hours. They might as well be in the military. If we think about how submissive and robotic children have to be during school, it kind of makes me wonder what they would be like as adults if they weren't so robotic and had a mind and spirit of their own.

But guess what? None of it Matters.

That's right – none of it matters. As human beings, we have the ability to take a look at life and see what works and what doesn't work for us. We can choose to accept society, religion, media and teachings of traditional schooling or we can choose not to. None of it matters because we have choices and all the possibilities that come from them. We can think and feel for ourselves, regardless of our stories and everything we see. One of my great teachers, Venus Brightstar, once said, "I may live on this Earth, with all these people but I am not of it." This basically means that although we live here in today's society, we really don't need to be part of it or anything else that doesn't feel right to our selves. Who is the Self now?

There's a difference between being Self-Centered and Centered on the Self. Self-Centered translates to not caring for anyone but yourself and centered on the self means taking a look at who you really are, within. With everything that we see, hear, smell, feel and experience in other ways, we are removed further and further away from our true self. The self that came into this world with a purpose, a passion and a beautiful beingness. That beautiful self is buried so deep under shame, hate, doubt, dark secrets, fear and illusions that it rarely sees the light of day.

Society, religion, media, school, the past or the future really don't matter to the True Self. They only matter to the Ego and Mind, which we as human beings are neither ego nor mind. We are souls, spirits and beings of a much less complicated essence. Our essence is pure energy which vibrates at a high frequency when the True Self can live freely. Now don't get me wrong, I have nothing against society, religion, media or education. It's the distorted rules, false ideas, self-hating mentality and the judgmental views they have on people that I choose not to be part of. I was once part of it all, a young girl sitting in church, hating myself because of the feelings I had for other girls. Confused as to who would love me for being so different from the girls on the magazines because I chose to listen to old Mexican music and paint the night away while drinking a bottle of Tequila for some inspiration.

All I'm saying is that what we think matters, really doesn't. Not our baggage or what people have to say about it matter. Our true self, our essence, our love, our spirit matters. We matter.

Pain Matters

by Gina Kramer

What is pain? Where does it come from? What causes it? Is mental and emotional pain as important or as painful as physical pain? Can mental and emotional pain manifest into physical pain? If you can't see it, does it really exist?

Pain is actually defined as: physical, mental or emotional distress, suffering or torment. It can come from nearly anything – from stubbing your toe to angry words that are exchanged. Pain is caused by receptors in the body sending signals to the brain and chemicals being released. Mental, emotional and physical pain are all equally important. Yes, mental and emotional pain can manifest into physical pain. Yes, it can exist even if there isn't a physical injury or explanation for it.

So then does your pain matter? How much does it

matter? Can you control how it affects you and your life? Are there steps you can take to limit the affects? Yes, your pain matters. There isn't any one answer for the rest of these questions. The answers vary as much as the person experiencing the pain. Each person processes pain differently, so it affects everyone in different way. So it's important that each person recognize and process their pain in their own way. Only in that way can they have some control over the affects pain has in their lives.

Pain comes in many forms and can be difficult to explain or pinpoint. The medical world classifies pain as acute or chronic and then defines it further into more categories. They also use many ways to measure the pain but since each person experiences pain in a different way, is any measurement valid? Is all of that really important? Yes, it is if you are dealing with it from a medical standpoint. What if you are dealing with pain that isn't necessarily a medical condition or pain that the medical community doesn't know how to deal with? What if the person prefers to deal with it in some way other than prescription drugs? Is it then important to measure it or simply acknowledge it? I'm sure there are many varying thoughts on this. My reasoning is this – it's only important that the person is feeling pain. If they have exhausted the medical search and nothing can be found or if the medical world has no real solution to the pain, then it is necessary to think outside of the box and realize there may be another way to deal with it.

If someone is experiencing emotional or mental pain and they choose to ignore it, it may eventually manifest itself as physical pain. Paying attention to pain does not mean dwelling on it, it's simply important to recognize it and be aware of how it affects us. It affects who we are, who we become, how we deal with life and how we deal with other people. The pain you feel may offer insights into where you are in your life, what is holding you there and what needs to happen to help you move forward.

There are many things that people say about pain. One of the favorites is, "Pain is weakness leaving the body." Because pain doesn't necessarily have an outward manifestation, it can be difficult for other people to identify with or recognize and they seem to feel the need to minimize it. Just because someone can't see it, doesn't mean it isn't real. Since pain can't always be seen or measured, people tend to minimize it saying things such as, "Just brush it off. You'll be alright," or "It only hurts for a little while," or "It's a long way from your heart" or the ever popular, "It's all in your head." While all of these may be true of some pain or in some cases, when someone minimizes your pain it can then cause more emotional pain because you feel as if no one is listening and you can't find an answer. The stress caused from that thought process may cause more physical pain and then it becomes a vicious cycle.

Pain is never fun to experience. It is however, part of life so by learning from it we can move through it more quickly and the pain goes away more quickly. In general, it is true that we learn more through pain than from pleasure which may be why really important lessons are often times very painful. We, as a human race, tend to dwell on painful situations more so than things we find pleasurable. So even though it isn't pleasant, there is almost always a lesson to be learned from pain. With that being said, it's important to realize pain has a purpose and there is a lesson to be learned from it. Your pain matters and should never be ignored. Experience the pain. Pay attention to the pain. Take note of when you feel it, how you feel it and where you feel it. Find the lesson in it and move through it.

Pain affects every part of our lives. It has an impact on our jobs, our health, emotional state, our overall well-being and our relationships. Visible signs of pain, while difficult to deal with, are more easily accepted by those around us. They can see the injury or the wound and that helps people understand the pain. When the pain comes from an invisible source, i.e. PTSD, Fibromyalgia, Lupus, emotional trauma or a long list of other painful conditions, it is much more difficult for others to understand. How can something hurt when there is no outward signs? They ask questions like, "How can someone look fine, healthy and functioning and still be in debilitating pain?" or "If there is no medical reason, how can it hurt that much?" When they can't see the cause of the pain, they begin to think various things such as; the pain is being used as an excuse, the person is lazy, they are just feeling sorry for themselves, they want attention or maybe there is something wrong with the person mentally. When someone is in severe pain with no outward appearance or "proof" and the people they care about begin to question if the pain actually exists, it often causes the person in pain to hide their pain even more. They then do their best not to show it and to push through it. In the process of hiding the pain, oftentimes burying it deep within themselves, they cause themselves more pain. What started out as severe physical pain then becomes emotional pain or begins to manifest itself in other physical ways. What was emotional pain becomes deepened pain or it may manifest as a physical pain as well. Either type of pain when ignored may lead to depression.

Because pain affects the person experiencing it and all those who interact with them, it can be difficult to process and move past. It is extremely important for the person in pain to acknowledge it and find a way to express it. Hiding it can only compound the problem. While recognizing the pain may not decrease it, it does give the person experiencing it the opportunity to work through it. Expressing it opens up the mind and the person's ability to work through it mentally and emotionally. Bringing things into the light often makes them appear smaller than initially believed. It's important to give people the opportunity to express how they are feeling, how the pain feels and how it makes them feel. Otherwise, they might think they need to hide it. Opening all of that up to the light helps them process the pain, their thoughts and emotions. It also helps them find a better way to deal with the people in their lives, their doubts and questions.

The pain that is currently experienced may be from something recent or it may be something buried in the past. Either way, it's important to acknowledge it. It may not be necessary to delve into the past and rehash all of your experiences to accept them and learn from them. It is however necessary to recognize the pain and acknowledge it. By admitting the pain exists, acknowledging it and accepting it, it is possible to learn from it, find solutions to it and move through it. That pain may serve several purposes. It may be a warning us to health issues. It may give us insight to past issues that are still affecting our lives now. It may show you what is holding you where you are currently in your life.

It's time to open up and express who you are. What makes you who you are? How do you feel about who you are and where you are in your life? How does what others in your life think makes you feel? How is your pain affecting your life? Do you need to change things? If so, what can you change? How you can change it? What steps do you need to take? What control can you take over your pain and how will you allow it to affect you? It's also important to understand your pain does matter...never let anyone tell you otherwise.

Positivity Matters

by Craig "Fett" Fetterolf

If you've become frustrated and discouraged with
how negative our society seems to have become,
there's something you can do about it right now –
not just for yourself, but for our culture and the
world at large. I've found a very tangible way to
deal with (and counter) negativity that I call my
"sphere of influence" approach. The gist of it is
quite simple: the only things we really have
immediate control or influence over are the people
and situations that we deal with directly and on a
daily basis. That's our own, personal sphere of
influence. If we focus positive energy on those
people and situations in our sphere, we can have a
profound effect on them. Then, if the people in our
sphere do the same with their own spheres, that
focused positivity spreads extremely quickly
throughout our culture – and the rest of the world.
It's sort of a new spin on the six degrees of

separation idea.

If you're wondering if this concept can really work, I'm proof that it does. Many years ago, I worked at General Electric. I had been working there for a long time, had done quite well and had developed a reputation for the quality of my work and for getting things done. But as a side-effect of having been there so long, I was also quite influenced by the corporate/office culture and had gotten pretty cynical. I had refined that cynicism into an irreverent, maverick personality that my co-workers admired, because I was always the guy who would bring up the "hard issues" and say the things that no one else was comfortable saying. Sometimes that smart-ass approach could be useful when things weren't moving forward or tough areas needed to be addressed. But my attitude and behavior also had a downside that I didn't see: they spread cynicism and negativity among my co-workers.

One day, I was on a video conference call with Headquarters. My boss was on the other end of the call with several managers from other departments at HQ, and I was with my co-workers in a conference room at the local office. I played my usual role of "bringing up the hard stuff" and asking the cynical questions on behalf of my work group. The problem was, that wasn't the point of the meeting. The point was to find common ground, work on solutions to problems, and help the project move forward. At the end of the meeting, my co-workers patted me on the back for having played the "heavy," and I thought pretty highly of myself. That was on a Friday afternoon.

The following Monday, as I arrived at the office, my boss confronted me in the hallway: "Into my office – NOW!" For the next half hour, my boss proceeded to "rip me a new one," explaining that my behavior in the previous Friday's meeting was not only inappropriate, but unacceptable. I got very defensive, telling him that I was just "doing my job" and playing the role that was expected of me as a long-term, experienced employee. He explained to me that I wasn't getting the point: It wasn't just that I had made myself and my co-workers look bad to the rest of the managers on the other end of the conference call; the real issue was that, as a senior employee, I was having a strong impact on the attitudes and behavior of those around me – especially the newer employees. He explained that they learned how to think and behave from me, so if I thought and behaved negatively, so would they. I resisted, telling him that results were what mattered most, not personalities. He wouldn't back down, and made it clear to me that, if I didn't take what he said to heart and start behaving differently, I would no longer be welcome in his group.

I went home later that day huffing and puffing about the whole situation and complaining about it to my wife, but at some point, for reasons I still don't comprehend, I started to see my boss's words as a challenge. Eventually, I decided to do a little experiment: For the following six months, I would consciously alter my thoughts and behavior around my co-workers, focusing only on the positive, and observe what happened. To my surprise – shock, actually – through only a change in my own behavior, *everything* about my group and the office environment changed. Everyone became more positive, and more things got done. We all actually started to have *fun* at work. By the end of the six months, my nickname at the office had even changed to the "Perky Little Turkey!" The positivity truly was contagious. I had simply set the tone, and my co-workers had followed.

I had another office-related experienced at General Electric that proved how much positivity – in this case, *persistent* positivity – can change people in our sphere of influence. There was a woman at the office named Brenda that everybody hated to work with. She was cold, brash, impatient and downright rude to pretty much anyone as a matter of course. Everyone wanted to avoid her, but unfortunately, she held a position that guaranteed that people would have to deal with her fairly frequently. The first time I met Brenda, she treated me the same way she treated everyone else: tersely and grumpily. I was required to work with her on several more occasions, and got pretty much the same reception from her every time. But it just didn't bother me. Instead of responding in kind (which is our first instinct when people are rude to us), I refused to be sucked into her vibe, so I simply smiled and greeted her as positively as I could, as if she hadn't treated me negatively at all.

Over many months – perhaps even a couple of years – I continued this dynamic with Brenda; she would be rude to me, and I would simply "nice" her back, every time. Then one day, out of the blue, it happened: Brenda "woke up" and realized that someone was being kind to her – not just once in a while, but *every* time. From that point onward, Brenda warmed up to me considerably, and eventually, she was just as positive to me as I was to her, and just couldn't do enough for me whenever I asked her for anything. She was a hard nut to crack, but even she could be cracked eventually, as I believe most negative people can. Ever since that lesson I learned with Brenda years ago, I've made a point of responding in reverse whenever people are negative toward me. And the more negative they are, the harder I push back with niceness. And just like Brenda, they eventually come around. The technique has served me so well for so many years that I actually have a term for it: "doing a Brenda on someone." If you have any "Brendas" in your life, try this technique out on them and see what happens. It might take a few tries and you might not get results overnight, but I'm confident that your experience will eventually be just like mine.

I experienced another example of the power of positivity in a motivational tape series by Tony Robbins many years ago. In one segment, Tony conducted an exercise that you can do yourself: Look around the room you are in, and while closely observing your surroundings, make a mental note of everything in the room that's colored brown. Really concentrate on the process, and when you've noted everything that's brown, close your eyes. Then, try to remember anything in the room that's *green*. I can guarantee you won't be able to do it. I've done this exercise with people I know many times, and it's uncanny how consistent the results are. This phenomenon goes by many names, most generally the Law of Attraction, but the point Tony Robbins was making was that if you focus on the "brown stuff" in life, that's what you'll see, and get more of. On the other hand, if you focus on the "greens and blues" of life, then *that's* what you'll see and get more of. It's just how our brains – and the universe – work.

My experiences at General Electric changed my life, but more important, I saw first-hand that they changed the lives of the people around me. And in turn, I believe it also changed the lives of the people around them – in their own spheres of influence. Since then, I've never looked back, and have made it a point of trying to be a positive person to everyone I come in contact with, from friends and family, to co-workers, to clients, to the clerk at the grocery store. And every time I do, I think about the impact it's having on them, and indirectly, on the people in their own lives. Imagine the snowball effect we can have on the world when we all use the sphere-of-influence or blues-and-greens approaches to life. Talk about going viral! I've seen firsthand that positivity doesn't just matter, it *changes lives*!

Self-Recovery Matters

by Nichole Terry

One of the most incredible things about this world is the concurrent presence and expression of Universal spirit through the various people who reside here. Each one of us is a powerful and potent manifestation of the Divine's complete personality and character. However, as the daily requirements of work, family and financial responsibilities fight for our attention, we may forget our precious uniqueness and individuality thus becoming drawn into the repetitive demands of societal conformity and conventionality. This results in the stifling of individual goals and abandonment of our unique purposes, passions and divine destiny which are to be enjoyed and flaunted during our time here on Earth. Accordingly, it is critical for us to continue to remind ourselves of who we are through self-recovery which can be obtained through enjoyment of the small blessings we experience every day, re-engaging in our talents and passions that we have neglected and maintaining this self-recovery through daily self-care and promotion.

What is Self-Recovery?

Many of us have not taken the time to preserve or acknowledge our original passions, desires and goals. We have become intricately overwhelmed and weighed down by the daily obligations of adulthood, and though these responsibilities are important, we have forgotten how self-promotion and self-love are equally critical for maintaining a healthy and balanced life. When the realization of self-loss is obtained, self-recovery must subsequently take place. Self-recovery is the revitalization of self through promotion of individual goals and desires despite current circumstances. It takes place when we remember and appreciate how incredibly unique and precious we are and give ourselves the attention and awareness that we have deserved every day of our lives. Self-recovery can be attained through several means. I am sharing two of my favorites: enjoyment of the small things and pursuit of individual passions and talents.

Recover Self through Enjoyment of the Small Things

When this earthly journey first commences, our innate childlike curiosity and inquisitiveness is the driving force behind our individual growth and development of our unique talents and God-given abilities. As a child, the world is a brand new, mysterious and exciting place where every question is followed by another question and every day provides us with new experiences and joys that we are not afraid to confront in or own exceptional ways. During our youth, our talents are new and explored, and creativity, imagination and dreaming is encouraged and allowed for. As children, we enjoy the small things. We play without self-consciousness, run without counting calories and jump without asking, "How high?" This is a time of spiritual freedom where our true selves are evident and present in the world, and we are free to experience life through the joy of merely living.

As adults, we do not always enjoy the world as we used to as children. Of course, our responsibilities grow and our obligations change but we don't realize the importance of taking the time to enjoy and celebrate our world as we did once before. When is the last time we enjoyed a walk in the park without a pedometer because we just had to count our steps or swung on a swing without counting it as exercise because the doctor said we have to get in 30 minutes a day? Life is to be enjoyed and every day we are alive, we should take the time to notice and appreciate the small wonders of this world. These little wonders that we took note of as children are what made childhood so precious and enjoyable. They can perform the same magic in our adult lives as well.

Recover Self through Diligent Pursuit of Individual Passions and Talents

What would you do for free? What do you enjoy doing so much that there is no amount of money that you would accept in exchange for doing it? The famous saying goes, "If you do what you love, you will never work a day in your life." This could not be a more accurate statement. It is apparent that the importance of currency is no doubt stressed in our society. We are judged based on how much money we make, our credit score and what possessions we own. However, these material items rarely bring long-lasting or ongoing fulfillment. The reason for this is that these tangible possessions are usually obtained through an attempt to be noticed by others and typically have nothing to do with us. For example, you felt pride when your business associates complimented your car, when your mother swooned over your expensive home, and your friends adored your brand new Louis Vuitton bag. However, after they finish complimenting you, you are left with the same unrewarding lifestyle that you were leading before because despite having these various things, you are plagued with this ongoing feeling of unfulfillment – as if something is missing from your life.

One of the easiest ways to alleviate these feelings of unfulfillment is to simply do what you love. Several of us are unhappy in our jobs or our careers. I'm not suggesting that you quit your job and risk a move into the streets. I'm suggesting a reevaluation of your passions and your goals with the intention of reigniting them. If you are not happy with your current situation, the best thing to do is work to change it. However, make sure that this change encompasses the things that bring you the most passion and excitement. If changing careers is not an option, then make an attempt to make time for what you love every day or at least a couple of times throughout the week. By doing this, you are recovering your true self and taking the time to enjoy your real authenticity.

Self-Care and Self-Promotion

Self-recovery can be attained even though demands of everyday life are vast and extensive. If self-recovery is not maintained, this can result in abandonment of individual needs, desires, goals and progression. When this occurs, several of us can become so engrossed in the expectations of society and culture that we completely desert our basic personal needs. Some of these needs include receiving and giving unconditional love, resting our spirits and minds and attending to our hearts desires. As a result of forgetting these needs, some of us commit to harmful and abusive relationships, depend on anti-depressants and psychotropics to merely get out of bed, or face our death beds with intense regrets for how our lives should have been. In order to work to maintain the efforts of self-recovery, it is crucial that we engage in daily self-care and promotional practices that keep our dreams, passions and life goals fresh in our minds. Below is a list of simple ways that we can include self-care and promotion in our busy, daily schedules:

Celebrate the little things.

We always take the time to commemorate the big things in life. However, the little accomplishments get overlooked. Make a note to celebrate all of the small pleasures and successes in your life. Giving attention to the smaller details allow you to appreciate yourself more as they tend to occur more than the larger accomplishments.

Thank yourself for completing everyday responsibilities.

Paying bills never seemed fun before now! Meeting your everyday responsibilities is a statement to your ability to care for yourself and others around you. Accordingly, you should appreciate the time and attention that you give to your own needs and value your everyday blessings. You have a vehicle to meet your needs so pay your car note with a smile. You have a roof over your head, so handover your rent or mortgage with a grin. Life is to be enjoyed, so take pleasure in every bit of it.

Take five minutes to close your eyes.

My mother is a wise woman and always has a good bit of advice for my recurring life issues. Once upon telling her how overwhelmed I was with all of my various responsibilities, she stated that I needed to take time to shut out life and relax every day. You might be thinking, "Who has the time?" Her response was, "Even if it's five minutes, it's better than nothing." My mother is correct. Despite the craziness of everyday life, it is incredibly important to take time to stop and mentally detach from the day and relax your mind, spirit and body. These five minutes can be experienced at any time of day in any place. All that you need is to calm your mind and to detach your mind in order to allow for the recuperation necessary to revitalize and rejuvenate your energy and thus balance the demands of life and your individual passions and goals.

Our individuality was handed to us by the Divine upon birth. Through that individuality, we have incredible talents and abilities that make us who we are. However, we forget these talents as we become engrossed in our everyday responsibilities and obligations. This is why self-recovery is so critical. Through self-recovery, we can regain ourselves through giving attention to our original desires and passions through re-engaging in activities we love and taking the time to enjoy the small blessings that make up our lives. Through self-recovery, we can now enjoy and promote our precious individuality given to us by the Divine and bless ourselves, our loved ones and the world around us with the very best of who we truly are.

Spirit Matters

by Megan Johnson Rox

I once had a student ask, "What happens when you listen to your gut instinct and it leads you to a bad/wrong decision?" I answered this in two parts. First, your spirit is never wrong! It takes practice to learn to distinguish your ego from your spirit. Second, how do you know it was a bad/wrong decision? Our spirit will always lead us down the path we are meant to go down, but sometimes, we need to learn certain things to progress, and those lessons are not always learned the easy way.

Following your spirit is not always easy. However, doing so usually prevents you from making a mistake that is even more difficult to recover from. We always learn from mistakes, but wouldn't it be nice if we had less of them? Life is so much easier when you trust your gut instinct. Gut instincts (or some call it intuition) are your spirit trying to guide you. My idea of spirit is not based in religion but rather that it's the soul that is in all of us, no matter what religion we are or aren't.

It's not always so simple to just follow your spirit or gut instincts. The problem comes when you follow what you think is your spirit giving you guidance but it's really your ego. To simplify it, the ego is your mind. The problem with the ego/mind is that it bases decisions on a set of rules/norms/guidelines that society and our parents/friends have told us is right. These rules/norms/guidelines about what is "rational/realistic/normal/logical" are so ingrained in us that they become our core beliefs and values and we don't even realize what they are anymore but they still subconsciously govern our decisions. When we use snap judgments, we are using these "rules". Often, it feels like our gut instinct, but is really not. This is why it's very important to take an inventory of our beliefs and values on everything.

It takes time to learn how to distinguish between your spirit and your ego. It's a skill that you need to develop and practice. It's hard to tell if what pops into your head is a thought from your ego/mind or a message from spirit. Usually, when you analyze something in your mind (or in my case, overanalyze), you're using your ego to make your decision. Usually, the instant feeling you have about something is your spirit's guidance. Spirit communicates through 'feeling', not thinking. You may think, it's not realistic or good to go about your life based on just feeling or gut instincts, but I can attest, after several years of trying this, that this IS the best way. That's not to say you don't need to use your mind to try to understand the message if it's vague or comes in an unusual package (seeing something that makes you think about someone for some reason, for example) or seems contrary to "popular belief", aka, societal norms or what has always happened in this situation for others. I hear people use this last one all the time. I'm too old to fulfill my dream because I rarely see people starting out at my age getting successful at this. Or, most people starting new businesses lose money the first few months, so I don't expect to. Or, I won't be able to find a job I like that has both the flexibility and freedom of schedule AND pays well. Remember, your path is not like anyone else's. Everyone has such unique, individual paths in life that you can't possibly compare yours to anyone else's path. So, what is not possible for someone else can be entirely possible for you and vice versa.

Every time I do NOT follow my spirit's guidance, it ends badly. However, following your spirit's guidance is often easier said than done. What makes it more difficult is when your spirit's guidance goes against the "rules/norms" ingrained in our thought and behavior patterns and our ego.

Let Your Spirit Take the Driver's Seat

Listen to your spirit and live your life from its guidance. It will never lead you wrong. I'm sure we've all had moments where we get inner guidance to do something but don't follow it and it ends up badly.

I have. For example, I was editing a paper and a thought popped into my head (this is how your spirit often guides you) that I should do a "save as" – a newer version to leave the content of the older version I was working on before I cut too much out of it. I pondered it for a second but my ego quickly dismissed it and I remember thinking, "Oh, I don't need any of that old content that I'm cutting out. I don't need to do a 'save as'." Guess what happened? Five minutes later, I was cutting a big section to paste it somewhere else in the document and forgot to paste it back in before I cut something else and the whole section was lost.

I'll give you another story. My husband and I were in Paris and were going to take a train to

Switzerland. We had an early morning train and figured we'd just take the subway. My husband had a strong feeling we should take a cab instead but because he had every reason to believe taking the subway would work fine (even though it would take longer) and was the cheaper option, that's what we did. Well, he learned the hard way not to dismiss his gut instincts. The subway train stopped in mid-tunnel for some reason and that delay caused us to miss our train to Switzerland.

So, even those of us who can recognize when our spirit is trying to guide us fall prey to the power of the ego to "rationalize" it away. It's something I practice every day. Your spiritual guidance will become louder and more obvious the more you practice. The problem is most of us filter our guidance/gut instincts through the belief system of our egos and if the instinct doesn't seem to make sense based on your current belief system, we don't follow it.

Your Spirit Is the Best Decision-Maker

So, you may be thinking, that's great if you can distinguish between your spirit and your ego, but what if you can't? How do you know if a feeling is coming from the ego or the spirit? This can be tricky because for someone who has cut themselves off from their spirit, e.g., someone who lives in and makes decisions from fear, their first feeling might be fear. Or pessimists who are always skeptical about everything and assume the worst are living from ego. You know exactly if something is coming from your ego if it is based in fear. That's not to say your spirit will guide you against doing something. If you feel something you think may be a gut instinct but aren't sure, stop and analyze it. You have to really be honest with yourself here. Is it possibly based on a deeper fear of something? If so, then it's coming from your ego. If the decision feels good to you (on a physical level, not rational/logical level), it's from your spirit.

I say physical level because our bodies speak to us but many of us aren't listening. I think most people don't recognize subtle things their bodies do that are an expression of their emotions. I often don't realize I'm clenching my jaw or picking my nails when I'm in stressful, uncertain or fearful situations. The first part of my body to feel badly is my stomach when I'm sad, upset, angry, scared or stressed. This is a topic that deserves its own book, but I just wanted to bring it up because if we listen to our bodies more, we can more easily distinguish between feelings or thoughts that are from the spirit or the ego. Not surprisingly, those who let their spirit take the driver's seat in their life usually have good mental and physical health.

It's natural to feel ego-based emotions like competition, jealousy, anger, guilt, judging others, etc...because our society has taught us it's ok to think or feel these things. But as you work to improve your spiritual/personal development, you pay attention to your thoughts and feelings and notice when you start to feel any ego-based emotion and can stop yourself right away and choose to feel compassion, forgiveness and love to yourself and others instead. Notice I said to yourself too. This is because we subconsciously project our own emotions/thoughts onto others. So when we are angry at someone for their behavior, we're subconsciously angry at ourselves for being the same way/thing. This goes for competitiveness too. If you judge others for being competitive, you are actually not liking that part of yourself that is competitive. When you can recognize this, you can forgive yourself for feeling competitive sometimes and then forgive others for their competitiveness. Same goes for any emotion. In the path to spiritual development (and enlightenment), we are human and aren't perfect. We slip up sometimes (though less and less frequently and for shorter periods of time when we're really connected with our higher selves). We just need to forgive ourselves and others for not being perfect. Many spiritual teachers, including two of my favorites, Marianne Williamson and Wayne Dyer, and books such as The Course In Miracles, The Disappearance of the Universe by Gary Renard, as well as many religious texts of different religions, say that the key to happiness is to always practice compassion, forgiveness and love.

Those who have a close connection with spirit know that you can achieve anything your heart desires and that there is plenty of abundance to go around for everyone, AND that each person's path is so unique, you can't possibly compare your path to anyone else's. Also, if you realize that we're all connected anyway, there's no need to compare yourself to or compete with anyone.

As with any emotion that comes from the ego, if you allow yourself to continue feeling them, you are blocking yourself from being connected with your spirit or as some know it as - higher self/God/the universal life force/all that is. That's what will bring you guidance, ultimate peace, health, happiness and success.

Here are some ways to help you better connect with your spirit. The closer you are to it, the clearer the guidance will be and the faster you will get it. The more often you do these things too, the clearer it will be.

1. **MEDITATE:** This is the main way you get in touch with your spirit. It is also the most important. I'm sorry if you thought there was an easy way to do this "personal/spiritual development stuff" but there is not. I know people who groan when I suggest meditation because everyone thinks it's so hard and that they can't possibly do it well/right or have the discipline to continue doing it. While it can be difficult (my mind chatters more than any of yours I'll bet), as with anything, it gets easier with practice. Also, I wouldn't have been able to really get into it and keep it up if it weren't for taking a class. Just like

with exercise classes, it really helps when you have a teacher there pushing you to keep going even when you're frustrated and think you just can't do it. Once you're able to quiet your mind once, it gives you the encouragement/motivation to keep going. For some people (like me), taking a class is the only way to get started. There are lots of free guided meditations and podcasts online. I've recently discovered the easiest and also most powerful meditation. It's a mantra-based meditation and a teacher has to give you a personalized mantra to repeat in your mind as you meditate. I got mine from Deborah King but Deepak Chopra also has this type of meditation. The most well-known of this type is Transcendental Meditation. I highly recommend this mantra-based type of meditation. It's like a super-charged, super-power way to instantly connect with spirit. All of the spiritual teachers say it's very important to meditate every day. I do it 20 minutes every day and when I don't, I start to feel my ego creeping in (in the form of anxiety and/or stress). Other activities can be meditative such as yoga, walking, sitting in nature, dancing, music, etc. Doing any activity that feeds your soul is great. Meditation is like church for the soul.

2. **JOURNAL:** Take quiet time every day to jot down your thoughts and feelings of what happened that day. The spirit often speaks to us through our writing and for many, writing is a good way to get in touch with the soul. Don't be afraid. It can be scary to uncover old emotional trauma/garbage or issues but it's necessary for spiritual development (and ultimately becoming much happier!).

3. **ASK FOR GUIDANCE:** Your spirit, as well spiritual beings around us who want to help us, just needs to be asked. They will answer you, but sometimes it takes time to get the answer (sometimes days or weeks). You have to be patient. The answer will come to you (sometimes in unusual ways, so pay attention) if you are

regularly meditating and journaling. If you're not, it's just like prayer. If you pray but don't take time to be quiet and listen for the answer, what's the point?

There are other ways to be closer to your spirit - to be able to live/make decisions through spirit instead of ego - but these are three important, major ones to start with.

Good luck and have fun getting to know your spirit and making life easier on yourself (and much happier!).

Stress Matters

by L'Vereese Britten

What really matters to me is that we have survived as a human being for thousands of years only to come to a new millennium with the same thought patterns of disbelief in self and the awareness that we are not worthy of happiness unless we strive to have all monetary and material wealth at our fingertips. This has become the destination to happiness. We have come to the point of our evolution to want gain and power over others more than ever before. Politics, religions, governments, organizations, groups of people and races have become our world. Somewhere within our lives, there is a separation of people by status, sex or affiliation. We have become a civilization where morals have somehow seemed to silently disappear. Not the rules or laws of society that govern these things as moral, but the nudges and loving thoughts. The anxiety that comes when you know you made the wrong choice. These morals are the morals of truth.

We have come to a time and place where the greed of the ego's thoughts of gain and success have had many lose their lives, been wrongfully judged and persecuted for this gain. Generation after generation, some form of separation has occurred.

What matters is that in the year 2013, we still have not been able to see the oneness in each and every one of us. We have allowed our vision of our self to become distorted and blurred. Not only are we not able to see the true self, but we are also unable to see the (self) in others. We focus our time on judging others and putting ourselves through undaunted stress. Perceiving the life we are living as a tomb of doom. How many people do we know in our lives who are truly happy with what they have, who they are and where they're at in their lives.

Now, we have all been seeking to know the meaning of our lives. Knowing deep down inside that there is something more – something better. These nudges have been with us since we could remember. Each and everyone of us has experienced this at some time in our lives. That ache that just won't go away. So what is it? Why does it feel like you're rushed and running out of time? How many of us have tried watching every documentary, taking every workshop, reading numerous books and went from church to church – looking for someone to give us the answer we seek.

I know I have tried time after time, only to lose sight of where and what I was truly searching for. In years past, I have re-created myself, transforming my inner life, attempting to let God be God by appreciating who I truly was so I could live my life totally and wholly.

I had to step away from what others thought of me

which truly was a reflection of myself. That part of me that I did not want to admit lingered in the depths of my soul. During my time of self-reflection, I looked at the "man in the mirror" and was disgusted for everything I saw which was what I did not want to be.

So I went on a spiritual expedition to find the purpose of my life. One day, out of nowhere, Spirit answered and showed me. Our life represented divine love, and that <u>L</u>ove <u>I</u>s <u>F</u>or <u>E</u>ver. I sat and pondered this for awhile, and the more I thought about it, the more it made me stress because now I had even more questions.

I understood love, but I thought, "How can you enjoy love when life is truly a hell? How can we live stress-free in today's world?"

I've researched this thought for over a year. A little bit of knowledge was given to me – a nudge every once in a while. Every nudge I received to search deep. Bits and pieces of my truth were revealed, but to truly understand living stress-free, I needed to research and define stress.

Merriam-Webster defines the word stress as having physical, mental or emotional strain or tension. Stress is a state of unresolved tension, arising from the pressures and demands of our daily lives which targets each and every one of us. Stress becomes our hardship in life. Our deepest fears and insecurities. Presenting itself in our lives, first as negativity then as people and in situations that come to play in our life.

Now keep in mind, God did not promise us exemption from things that cause us stress. But we were all given the tools we need to enable us to live in such a way that these things will not hinder our growth.

So how do we know whether we are experiencing stress or not? Maybe you are and you're not aware of it. You may feel that what you are or have been experiencing is a normal function of life, but this experience of stress can cause a host of destruction in our lives.

This thing called stress, this affliction, produces a sense of anxiety, frustration, irritability and even depression. It creates a feeling of hopelessness and disillusionment which undermines our sense of purpose, direction and meaning in life. So many things can contribute to stressful living, especially in today's world:

Constant challenges and deadlines

The ever-changing state of our unstable world

Fear of uncertainties about our future

Failure to seek adequate rest and relaxation

Spiritual conflicts

Unresolved conflicts or emotions

These little things that, at the very moment we experience them, can prevent us from fulfilling our life's purpose or even hearing the inner voice of spirit.

This accumulated effect of long-standing stress causes dis-ease in our lives that will create an imbalance in the Chakras and eventually will cause disease in our bodies.

So what can we do to create a healthier happier life?

What is the wholeness behind our health? What is a healthier you?

Metaphysically speaking, our health could be defined as:

Healing Every Aspect To Our Lives Totally and Holistically

What do I mean by holistically?

Holistic is the belief that disease is a result of physical, emotional, social or environmental imbalance. This concept is the belief that all aspects of people's lives, include psychological, physical and social, should be taken in account and seen as a whole. Science is now understanding that the body, mind and spirit are all connected. An analogy of a human trinity could be defined as the body being a vehicle, the mind being our driver and the soul being a passenger.

A complete system synchronized in unity, which then completes us as human beings. So why do so many of us forget to maintain our vehicle? Why doesn't it matter to us? Why don't we tell the driver to take a driving break on long-distance drives? Why do we risk running our vehicles on an empty tank?

Through my self-discovery and the belief that I did

not want to live my life ill or indecisive, I promised myself that I would discover this love of life and the happiness that I felt I really deserved. A true Heaven on Earth. I discovered that with self-reflection and acceptance, I was worthy. I could see through the veil and realized that happiness was real. But it came from the internal part of me, and once I saw and felt this, my outer world changed.

So why does this matter? Why try and understand the true uniqueness of our beings? Why? So we are able to see that the value of our worth is so much more than what we perceive.

You do have a choice on how you live your life. You have a spiritual toolbox. So why should we try living our lives stress-free?

We have free will to choose happiness that allows divine love to flow through us.

This really matters. Living stress-free in today's world can give you greater awareness of the beautiful life we should be living. So let's finally start living life to the fullest. Start choosing to incorporate simple principles into your daily lives for stress-free living. I have nine suggestions you can choose to use in your life:

Daily Meditation: We can "allow" for a solution in any matter in our lives that may cause us stress. This will bring you rich fulfillment. The key is learning is to trust.

Dealing with Unresolved Conflicts: We must deal with all unresolved issues. Forgiveness gives us the compassion to love. Whatever conflicts that may be in your life, learn to deal with them as they come up. The longer you delay, the longer to heal from the outcome.

Manage Your Time: We must manage our time constructively so we can take the needed actions to change our situation. This involves pacing ourselves in such a way that we do not take on too much in a given time and understand our limitations.

Rest and Renewal: Take a day where you truly rest. No physical or mental work. Just do the things you like and the things that make you truly happy!

Healthy Eating Habits: Make a conscious effort to eat healthier. Eating healthy ensures that you will have more energy, feel better, lose weight and it ensures that your body is strong enough to fight off ailments and is capable of healing all illnesses.

Prayer: Release all that does not serve you daily. When you surrender, there is no anger or room for regret. You can truly forgive.

Visualization and Affirmations: Vision and affirm the life you want to live, and BELIEVE it!

<u>Gratitude:</u> THANK GOD daily for all that you have and all that you shall receive. Gratitude will make your manifestations a reality much quicker.

These steps have made me realize that when I choose to counteract negative feelings and thoughts with pure goodness, love and the thought that I am worthy, it is my right to be happy, healthy and loved, both individually and universally. Then and only then am I free. In love, flying free to pursue, dream and be the perfectly good, loving and beautiful Soul that I am. Then and only then will we be living in the now, truly living stress-free with greater awareness.

This truly matters.

Movement Matters

by Krystalyn Norton

Imagine, if you can...if you will...a flow. Think like water. Relax, let it flow through the pathways of your mind. The movement of matter is what we observe and we observe that matter moves. It moves in waves, in pulses. You are matter that moves and thus matter moves within you. Some of us move using maps, others with reckless abandon. Through three dimensions of x, y, z and then a fourth dimension of time, we move.

Time moves on. No matter, we have no power over that dimension. We are born into time, into a moment coming down the line and year after year, decade after decade, we live through the flow of time. Our choice here, then, is to flow with the movement of time in the present moment and seemingly, like time, move forward.

On the other hand, we have the power to look back and ask ourselves if we did all we could or did all we should.

That "should" is where we get hung up, a judgment of the self which needs no such accusations. Where and how do we feel this hang-up? In the body, in the mind, in the soul...we feel a weight. To let the passing of time wash away the weight, leaving lightness, ease some would call it. Letting only when "let," the flow is continuous and doesn't let up for anyone or anything. We get stuck on that thought of "should have" or "did" and it erodes from the inside out. "If I had only..." or "I could have..." Thoughts like these, of judgment and the past, arise. Lost in our own thoughts that swirl back around the same lesson time after time, not quite understanding, we stagnate. Piling up the corrosive thoughts, we push ourselves to the edge and like a dam made of judgment that holds back the raging waters, we eventually break if we are not willing to bend. To withstand the world, that's what it takes.

Held in place by fear, a social paralysis. A social paralysis of identity to hold you in place so you don't step out of line. Even within our own minds this paralysis takes hold, so we stand in our own way. Fear in our gut that holds us where we are, in stagnation, in insecurity. Intending on flow and yet loss of momentum keeps us from moving easily. That judgment, a being held, a state of being observed holds us up. Fear to trust the universe. To understand that it will be ok, better even, if we allow ourselves to be purified through vibrational manifestation and through the communication of our process. Our process of creativity moves us to manifest ideals. Creating with our words and our manifestation process, into the physical plain, facilitates our transformation. This openness to share allows for flow and thus gives us an outlet to keep it moving.

The sanskrit word for heart chakra, anahata literally translates to "unstruck" if you are struck with something like a stick. What might you do? Flinch, defend, take cover...a reactionary barrier to the transference of energy from the stick to you. What if that energy just moved through you like a ripple only stretching you a bit rather than impacting you bluntly? What if you received the world with openness and surrender? Your energy would be used to expand and live rather than defend and just survive.

So what does it mean to live? To get the fullest out of the life that you have received.

To find comfort within the body you have received as your vessel. This is our intention.

Intentional movement in the physical plane keeps the blood flowing, moving. The body is our most direct link to the physical world of motion. You can intend on being in a place at a time and thus you move the mass of molecules which is called the body from one place to another.

Self-realization is an expansive and uncovering process. After a few or many broken dams or broken dreams, for holding up the flow, we come to understand that to rid ourselves of the resistance is much less devastating. We ask why not forgiveness? Stop holding the breath. Then we breathe deep and long. We bring awareness to the stagnation and ask it to flow. Breath brings movement...movement is medicine, a means of healing, allowing blood to flow in and carry away the soup of emotion that resides in our being.

It dissolves the blockage, allowing space for welling up within us...a continuous emptying.

A shift of perspective thus opening two floodgates from head-to-toe and toe-to-head, if you will. Such allowance would be a practice of trust. Trusting of the universe, a willingness to listen, to be present, to surrender. A sitting with the stillness...the stillness that we know nothing about. The unknown, our ultimate perfection which we are always moving towards, the space between the particles, between the thoughts, is the unseen and the unobserved, thus the true.

The stars move in relation to where we are. Relation being motion between two points, a change in position and time. Allowing the constriction and the expansion to be in continuous flow as not to stagnate at any one point. Vibrating, pulsing something like the hours.

Circles we walk, to know ourselves, learning and relearning, layer after layer, after layer, uncovered in expansion. And created layer after layer in a symphony of color vibration.

Vibration...Need I say more?

Supernal Love Matters

by IAYAALIS Kali-Ma'at ELOAI

Okay. What? So...you are stating that
A SUPERNAL LOVE Matters.
Um...what is that again, please?

Well, it might be best to begin my declaration honoring SUPERNAL LOVE by quoting the Jamaican spiritual teacher or guru Anthony Paul Moo-Young, also known as Mooji, in which he states:

"To know what is LOVE...nobody can understand what is LOVE. Romantic LOVE is only an aspect. Children-Parent LOVE is only an aspect. LOVE for 'this and that' is only an aspect. You cannot pinpoint and say, 'Okay. It is this.' There is more space in not knowing than in apparent knowing. To know what is LOVE...nobody can understand what is LOVE."

I feel it's best to initiate with a quote like this and

in this way due to the fact that the overall meaning of this beautiful Life Principle we call LOVE still manages to somehow elude us all. And yet – it is so real. I mean, the biggest and brightest minds throughout time have never stopped discussing it or trying to figure it out.

The thought experiments of C.S. Lewis explored the nature of LOVE from a Christian perspective, highlighting the four distinct Greek words for LOVE: *Storge*, *Philia*, *Eros*, and *Agape*. These are words to describe different types of LOVE. To break it down in a very simple way: *Storge* is affection; *Philia* is friendship; *Eros* is romance; and *Agape* is unconditional LOVE. These are the basics. They are the most commonly accepted and understood types of LOVE.

Next, naturally, one may ask:

So…why does A SUPERNAL LOVE Matter?
and…what is a SUPERNAL LOVE?

(((sigh)))

And this is where my personal story begins...

What now seems like an entire lifetime ago was actually only about five years from this date, in which I was imprisoned in a self-created, hellacious nightmare of an existence. I was suffering under a dreadful diagnosis which modern medicine claims is an "incurable disease" called Multiple Sclerosis. My condition then was severe. I had experienced blindness due to optic neuritis three times already in each and in both eyes. The neuropathy that I had gone through had my brain erroneously reacting to it and my body tragically feeling the sensation of water as if it were the burning feeling of fire. At that time I was almost completely bedridden and in constant chronic pain. The state of my physical health was so excruciatingly depleted that it was a challenge to sit, stand, or walk without assistance.

Prescribing precarious pharmaceuticals and

predicting paralysis from the waist down at best, my doctors became the best outspoken soothsayers over my life. In the beginning I suppose I felt a sense of refuge under all their medical expertise and I did everything they commanded, only my health seemed to just get worse – and quickly. After a while, I really didn't know what to do. I was desperate. I was in darkness, and I knew Death was coming for me.

It was as if suddenly my entire existence had come to a screeching halt, and there I was – tired and tormented at a sad catastrophic crossroads of destiny...and no one was in that limbo – but ME.

A choice had to be made.
Was I going to flee or was I going to fight?
Was I going to live or was I going to die?

Ultimately, I did neither.

I was honestly too tired to fight and too fatigued to

flee, so I remained helplessly stationary in my limbo at the crossroads. In that darkest hour I was alone. I was broken. There was nothing left. So I surrendered to the nothing that was there. I allowed it to swallow me whole. In that space I felt all the pain and all the sorrow and held myself silently present in the face of all my fears.

In the midst of all that reckoning, an abrupt revelation came.

Suddenly, I realized I absolutely knew nothing – not a thing.

Well, I take that back. I did know there was a power Higher than me. I was not absolute on what the name of that power was, or even if that mysterious force greater than me was even vested enough in my existence to truly be concerned as to whether I lived or died. However, I did know there was something beyond me that existed...and it was then that I managed enough courage, and with *everything* in my being, to sincerely ask whatever it was that was out there for help.

Help came.

Now, I was raised by a good family in a house of strict and conventional religious principles. My parents are Catholic and are still very devoted followers of Christianity. However, I have personally been more open-minded and free-thinking my entire life. Therefore, I knew and was associated with many people of all different practices of faith. So when a dear friend of mine, who was quite adept in the mysteries of traditional African religion, agreed to "go to the mat" and consult the oracle of D'Ifa on my behalf, it was, admittedly, a different approach – but not so far-stretched for me. Not only that, but – what did I have to lose?

After consulting the oracle, my friend explained to me that The Great Mothers, Iyami, were present and expressed a desire to come to my aid. Of course, at that time I didn't totally understand what all that meant, but getting some kind of real help sounded great. I was instructed to simply persevere and pray, to keep my faith and know that help from the heavens was soon coming.

The definition of the word SUPERNAL is: of or relating to the sky or the heavens; of exceptional quality or extent. Synonyms for the word SUPERNAL are: celestial, divine, godlike. Now, I have known all kinds of LOVE before in my life – the LOVE of family, friends, and lovers, both conditional and unconditional. And yet, it is a SUPERNAL LOVE that completely changed my entire life for the better.

After talking to my friend and listening to her tell me about how The Great Mothers were sending me help from the heavens, I recall feeling a bit more uplifted and hopeful by her words, but tired. So I decided to go to sleep; only this time, I chose to focus on keeping my mind on something more prayerful and positive while I slumbered. I was hoping the words would somehow filter in my mind and entrain my subconscious in some kind of miraculous way. I couldn't read at the time because my vision was deeply affected by the various symptoms of optic neuritis and the whirling sense of vertigo in my head, so I chose to listen to an audio book instead. I chose to listen to *A Course in Miracles.*

I remember I fell into a deep dream state. In my dream I was seated at a desk at the front of a large classroom. The man, who my mind conjured up to be behind the voice of the audio book, was looking at me directly and teaching me.

"This is a course in miracles...The course does not aim at teaching the meaning of LOVE, for that is beyond what can be taught. It does aim, however, at removing the blocks to the awareness of LOVE'S presence, which is your natural inheritance. The

opposite of LOVE is fear, but what is all-encompassing can have no opposite.

This course can therefore be summed up very simply in this way:

Nothing real can be threatened.
Nothing unreal exists.

Herein lies the peace of God."

I don't recall many of the interesting little details of my dream. I just know that when I woke up from my slumber, I felt at peace. I felt refreshed. I felt renewed.

Honestly, it was as if my entire perspective somehow flipped into something wonderful and positive and highly vibrational. Not only that, the actual everyday events in my life also somehow flipped into something wonderful and positive and highly vibrational. I'm not referring to a mere gradual change either. I am testifying to an *immediate* change.

It was actually kind of eerie at first. It was almost like I was hearing the theme song to Rod Serling's classic television series, *The Twilight Zone,* play in the ethereal background of my mind. I silently mused to myself and thought, *"My mind is playing tricks on me – right?"* I couldn't quite grasp what had happened. All I knew was that my personal outlook upon my whole life had suddenly and magically transformed. Just as magically, the events in my life seemed to shift as well – for the *better.*

Please, understand that not all the major changes in my life, especially regarding my physical health, were immediate. Not all the modifications to my world were extreme. Some revolutions were more subtle than others. The evolutionary processes of some transformations in my life and in my being are even *still* in progress. But a significant change did happen.

Okay. So... what changed exactly?

My spirit changed. My awareness changed. My state of mind changed.

Gradually, my thoughts began to shift from a more negative focus to a more positive one. And thoughts *do* become things – so more positive things started manifesting in my life.

I went from hospital MRI scans showing over 50 active legions or scar tissue on my brain to, just a few years later, an MRI showing zero active legions on my brain. My relationship with my family transformed from what was nearly nonexistent, apathetic and dysfunctional to healthy, respectful, close and involved. I evolved from a negative, fearful, proud, angry and hurt soul to a more humble being enthusiastically ready to share her light and her LOVE to All.

I know LOVE to be a beautiful and an exceptional Life Principle. I know it to be a very powerful force of nature. I am aware of the different types of LOVE as well. However, from my perspective and life experience, a SUPERNAL LOVE, a high, celestial, more divine quality of LOVE, is truly what matters.

Healing Touch Matters

by Donlee Likins

I am a Certified Holistic Coach specializing in Intuitive Wellness Coaching and Healing Touch in Nashville, Tennessee. In this chapter, I will be talking a little bit about what I do, why it matters, and how you can use it in your own life.

So, you're probably wondering, "What is Healing Touch?" Healing Touch is a nurturing, energetic therapy first developed in 1980 by Janet Mentgen, a registered nurse based in Lakeland, Colorado. HealingTouchProgram.com describes Mentgen as "an energetically sensitive nurse. Her drive was to deepen and expand the connection between nurses and their patients. She saw the positive effect of touch while using various energy techniques and modalities." Mentgen spent eight years developing her "healing touch" and sharing it by teaching continuing education classes for nurses. In 1988 Mentgen's research, application

and teaching of her method won her the Holistic
Nurse of the Year Award from the American
Holistic Nurses Association. After a year spent
formalizing her techniques, Mentgen created the
Healing Touch certificate program which was
sponsored through the American Holistic Nurses
Association (AHNA). Three years later her Healing
Touch program was certified through the AHNA.
Of Mentgen's modality, HealingTouchProgram.com
explains, "Healing Touch emphasizes
compassionate, heart-centered care in which the
provider and client are equal partners in
facilitating wholeness. Healing Touch restores
harmony, energy and balance within the human
energy system and supports the self-healing
process of becoming whole in body, mind, emotion
and spirit. Healing Touch complements
conventional health care and is used in
collaboration with other approaches to health and
healing."

Healing Touch allows me and other practitioners

to approach every person as an energetic being. As humans, we appear solid and whole but scientists have now proven what scholars and poets alike have been hypothesizing forever...we are energetic. For example, when you look at the human body, you see we are made up of skin and bone. You know we have organs and blood. A very simplified jump: skin is made up of cells; another jump: cells are made up of atoms. Ten years ago, science told us atoms were the building blocks of all life and that we couldn't get any smaller than that. They've since discovered that atoms are more or less a shell encasing energy waves. So the very basis of all existence is the same...energy. So why does this matter?

This matters because as energetic beings, we are susceptible to all other forms of energy. And since literally everything is energy, and because most of it we cannot see or do not consider (i.e. the air that fills a room, the air we breathe to live), we are totally missing a huge part of who we are. Think of a time you walked into a place -- be it at work, a grocery store, maybe a park -- and you felt like you had to turn around. "Bad vibes." Or you are hosting an event, like a birthday party, and someone walks in and the atmosphere in the room changes...you can tell that person is really angry. You can feel this person's anger. This is energy. So how can we use this in our daily lives?

Our energetic awareness plays a key role in our physical health. Janet Mentgen was able to perceive energetic patterns and grids. She used these patterns to help diagnose and treat a physical and/or emotional ailment by healing the energy system supporting it. For example, that anger we were talking about. First, think about how a toddler experiences anger. They get red in the face, they scream and cry, they flail their fists and feet all about, they stomp and kick, they shake. Their reaction to feeling anger is fully experienced and fully expressed. Now think about how you, an adult, might experience anger. We might not experience it at all, right? We're at work and our boss yells at us for something we had no control over -- what do we do? We talk ourselves out of it, or we shove it down and ignore it. That anger didn't go anywhere. We interrupted the process. That anger is still with us. Instead, we might get a headache, we might have an ulcer...so instead of manifesting physically as expression (what we call a tantrum, acting out our anger), it manifests physically. Anger often comes through as headaches, shoulder problems, upset stomach or acid reflux, just to name a few. Deeply repressed anger is most often seen in chronic conditions and diseases. We cannot change anger itself, but we can change its place in our lives.

This brings us to the law of the conservation of energy, which states that energy can neither be created nor destroyed, but can change form. Going back to our anger example, when anger is triggered or picked up in our system, if we do not do anything to exert or release that energy, it does not go anywhere. We simply accept and ignore it. This allows it to stay in our energy system and the longer it stays the more static it becomes, the more solid it becomes, the more physical it becomes. Energy like this can manifest in a variety of ways, and can cause physical and emotional upset in our body, mind, and/or spirit.

As an Intuitive Wellness Coach specializing in Healing Touch, I am able to meet with a client and help them assess their own energetic body. This allows us to work together in bringing harmony and balance to their world through deep relaxation techniques and insightful, intentional goal-setting.

First, we start with a pre-treatment energetic assessment. This is my first impression of the client as an energetic being. As a highly sensitive person, intuitive and empath, I am able to see the person's energy just as I see the person. I am also able to feel in my own being what my client might be experiencing mentally, emotionally, physically or spiritually. Back again to our anger example: I might immediately feel the anger in my own body, or I might see this person in my mind as very angry or sad. My teeth might clench or I might feel breathless, my neck might start hurting. All of these register to me in this moment as indicators for anger.

After the intuitive intake, I discuss with my client anything they would like to approach in our session. Depending upon what my client wants to address and based on the information I receive during the intuitive intake process, I decide which healing touch intervention might be needed. I have my client move to a comfortable position, preferably lying face up fully clothed on a massage table. (Healing Touch was developed by nurses, remember, so all of the intervention techniques were created to allow easy and effective treatments to patient's hospital beds.) Once my client is comfortably lying on the table, I reassess the energetic field while consulting my intuition and considering the client's goals. Then a course of action is taken.

The process of attuning to a client through Healing Touch allows the client to fall into a deep state of relaxation. Many clients fall asleep at this time. While the client is in that deep state, their energy opens up. Information becomes more easily accessible. So, while holding this space, the client's energy begins to "breathe". It expands and regulates itself. (This is why stress is so bad, by the way.) As the client's energy is regulating itself, still attuned, I am able to channel important information.

I then do a post-treatment energetic assessment where I am able to chart the differences in the client's energetic system. It is not uncommon for practitioners to see changes in the physical body as well. Posture, for example, or evenness in the length of the legs, or balance of the shoulders.

After this, I ground and close. This just means I help gently bring the client back into the conscious level and disconnect from their energy system. Often, the energy work done during a Healing Touch session continues in motion well after the session - "until the healing is done," my mentor always says. This goes back to the law of the conservation of energy. Once that healing energy pattern is put into motion, it cannot be stopped. It's a domino effect.

When the client comes off the table, we review the treatment. This allows clients time and space to reflect upon the period of supported relaxation and how this feels. Often clients are able to come to their own truths and gain clarity on their personal life situations and their overall well-being. Recurrent sessions can offer clients great relief and/or new insights that result in heightened awareness of their own desires and ways of being. This can also help clients to find support and belief within themselves.

This type of meditative "anti-work" is deeply personal and unique to each client and each session. My work as an Intuitive Wellness Coach is to facilitate and support my clients in achieving the optimal overall health and well-being so that they can flourish.

Art Matters

by Janay Moreland

In 2012, I sat down with my spirit-self and we had a conversation about our future. I had just been diagnosed with major depression and major anxiety. I was a mental health counselor so I knew what those terms meant. I realized that throughout the years of schedules, dates, past due notices, term papers and deadlines, that I had driven myself mad! I was worried about my future (Anxiety) and could not let go of my past (Depression). At this crossroad in my life, I was in stagnation. I was at the crossroad of life we sometimes come to when we feel powerless and without direction. Simply existing. This diagnosis awakened me to the reality that I had lost control of my mind and spirit.

In talking with my spirit-self, I realized that I needed to start making personal, emotional changes. I knew that I could not turn back time to happier days. Turning back the clock was not possible. However, I did not know how to move forward in optimism. I had discovered I had loss myself in the trenches of life.

I began to think back to a time when I was more balanced - to a time when I was more at peace with myself. When I could sit in a room by myself and be at peace. As a teen I was very social and active. I enjoyed being around people and my thoughts were optimistic and ambitious. At present I was *majorly depressed and majorly anxious.* WHAT HAPPENED TO ME?!

After my internal conference with my spirit-self I began to pray for a solution. A few weeks later I ran across some old drawings from high school I had filed away years ago before I went away to college. I was reminded of how much I used to love art and being creative. I had always had a passion for art. When I was 4, my kindergarten teacher asked me to draw a little girl holding a flower. The daycare ended up using the painting as the logo for our graduation event. I enrolled in a by mail art school in middle school. I drew all throughout high school and was in the advanced art class. I don't remember when I departed from my passion. I hadn't drawn or painted in 7 years!

This discovery sparked something within me. At that moment, I made a vow to rediscovered myself. I started rummaging through closets and drawers until I found my old set of pastels and charcoals. I sat down and began to draw the first thing I looked at, which was my left hand.

 I began drawing. This was the first time in a long time that I didn't hesitate before beginning a project. I didn't feel the need to plan. Everything within me was saying "just do it." It was the first time in a long time I felt free to be myself. Free to create without restriction. Free to let go of the outside world.

By the time I finished my drawing, I felt dizzy with a strong surge of energy. I felt like I had released something and had taken something in all at the same time. My mind felt very relaxed. All I wanted to do was draw another picture. My second drawing was of koi fish. After about two hours into my project, my carpet, jeans, and cats were covered in chalk dust. It was a frenzy of color and energy all over the room. I was happy! This is when I began to realize that ART MATTERS.

Art is a combination of many factors. Most important of these factors is that art is a creation. What is a creation? A creation is a thought. What is a thought? A thought is a spark of energy produced in the brain. This means that art is energy. Because others can view this art, art is the sharing of energy. Art allows us the ability to produce a universal language that can cross any culture or language. If art is energy and the body needs energy to function, then art can be viewed as an essential part of our life. Whether we are creating it or viewing it, art is important in our everyday lives.

Art is energy. This energy feeds into the mind, body and soul. If art provides us energy, this means art has the ability to balance out depleted or shuffled energy. On way this is made possible is through the elements of color. Colors emit energies that evoke emotions. They affect us physically and mentally. Reds make our muscles tense while blues relax them. The color of a crystal or a stone can give emphasis to its powers. For example, the calcite is a blue stone that is good for calming the body and encouraging inner stability and security. Red jasper activates circulation and helps weakness and exhaustion.

During my early days of rediscovery through art, I began to notice that certain paintings would make me feel energized mentally and physically while other paintings made me feel relaxed and even sluggish. I began to notice my environment as well.

My apartment was full of dark color. How could it harbor happiness? My bedroom was decorated black, my living room was decorated black and brown with a dark green couch. Everything around me was dark and gloomy. I would come home from a busy, high-strung, stressful job to a wo-mancave of darkness and despair. Talk about needing an interior decorator! I didn't have the money to redecorate so I decided to hang my paintings on my walls. I was able to create and stabilize my emotions while also establishing a mini art gallery. Not only that, I was surrounded by what made me connect to my spirit-self.

Theo Gimbel, author of *The Healing Energies of Colour*, states that we are bathed in color from our day of conception. Our food is bathed in color; our clothing; our environment. Color surrounds us daily. He says, "Color dominates our senses." We feel through color. In nature, color speaks. It confirms safety vs danger. Color influences our language. People can be "green with envy," having "the blues," or be "seeing red." In every aspect of our life's color and art surrounds us. ART MATTERS.

For about a year, I had a ritual where I would come home, jog in the neighborhood, paint, cook (create), and the rest of the night or do a fun or social activity. During this continued pattern, I began to realize that I was not happy with my job. Because I had become more in tune with my emotions through art, I had come to recognize things that bothered me and that weren't good for me. My spirit-self knew I was in the wrong environment to pursue my life purpose. I began to brainstorm on what my purpose could be in life. I wrote my ideas and passions down and came to the conclusion that I wanted to help people feel Joy. I felt that others should be able to get a glimpse of the release I had begun to experience through art. After a few months of networking, researching and planning, I quit my job, eventually became a certified Holistic Life Coach, and created a company that specialized in helping individuals heal emotionally through art, color, and creativity.

Art helped me to heal. It helped me to reconnect to my spirit-self and to hear her voice more clearly. She was lost in the shuffle of life stressors, deadlines, unexpected events, unmet expectations and emotional rollercoasters. Art brought her and I back together.

Art healed me.

Art, my first love.

This is why ART MATTERS.

Ahmisā Matters

by Katy Brandt

atha yoga anuśāsanam
> *Yoga Sutras*, I.1

"Now we come to yoga."

ahiṃsā pratiṣṭhāyāṃ tat-saṃnidhau vaira-tyāgaḥ
> *Yoga Sutras*, II.35

"When the yogi is grounded in the virtue of non-harming, all enmity is abandoned in his presence."

maitri-ādiṣu balāni
> *Yoga Sutras*, III.23

"By sticking to the principles of non-violence (Ahmisā), one acquires strength and power as well as friendliness."

As I sit down to write this, the United States, where I live, has just gone through a historic campaign to elect a new president. The campaign has been divisive and created a lot of animosity between people. The country is deeply divided and the chosen leaders are deeply disliked by a historic portion of the population. The end result was a surprise and is a deep disappointment to many. But the choice has been made and now we have to move on as a country and work for the good of all citizens.

So what does this have to do with wellness? Everything.

In order to be well, we need to feel safe, we need security, we need the basics of survival: food, shelter, water. Our governments are key in modern society to protecting these needs for individuals. And in order to govern there must be cooperation between people. In a world divided, how do we get there?

Personal wellness is where the journey begins and ends. For those of us who study yoga, we know there are secrets in the *Yoga Sutras* to guide us. And it is all about unity. 'Yoga' is translated as 'to yoke,' or to create unity within the self by fully integrating mind, body and spirit and then fully integrating with our world. If we can become accomplished as yogis, we accomplish this goal realizing the best that life has to offer to be whole as individuals and as members of society.

In yoga, we study the eight limbs as a path to wellness and enlightenment, starting with the Yamas. The Yamas are simply five principles of self-discipline. I like to think of them as the first five commandments of yoga. They are Ahimsā (non-violence), Satya (truth), Asteya (non-stealing), Brahmacharya (chastity), and Aprigrahā (non-greed).

I don't think it was an accident that when Patanjali took the time to record the basic tenets of yoga in the *Yoga Sutras* that the first principle he decided to lay down was the practice of Ahimsā. Non-violence, or non-harming, is so essential to our wellness as individuals and as members of society. Without it, we have chaos. Chaos is what many citizens in the United States are fearing today. There has been violence in the campaign we observed. There have been perceived calls to violence. And there is fear that the chosen leader will be quick to use violent actions. In short, we are not well. We are not connected within ourselves and to others. We have lost our way by not practicing our yoga.

So, what about this idea of Ahimsā, non-harming, in yoga? It sounds like it means we need to be kind to others and our earth. It seems to most to be an outward expression. And it is. But that is not the whole story.

How can we be non-harming outwardly when we continue to harm ourselves? In our daily lives, we continually do things to sabotage our own wellness. We work too many hours. We do not get enough sleep. We sacrifice time for ourselves in order to do things for others that are not appreciated. We do not eat like we should. The list goes on and on. And what is the result? A society of people who are barely functioning trying to keep up. We are tired and stressed. We are getting sick. Health care costs in Western society are skyrocketing. People are turning to prescription (and non-prescription) drugs to help them function. And it is just getting worse.

As we continue to neglect ourselves, we begin to neglect our society and our world. It is like a snowball. One small harm to ourselves builds into many and as we become unwell we start to lash out. Maybe that outward action is subtle.

Something as simple as walking past someone in need or failing to recycle when we can easily do it. It all builds into a population that is suffering. We see it every day.

As a yoga instructor, I talk about non-violence, or non-harming, a lot. Many of us walk into the practice of yoga because we think it will be a path to heal … something. Whether it is stress, a general sense of being off balance, or a physical ailment, we are hearing that yoga is a part of the solution. So we begin to explore. We have an idea that yoga will be good for us and that it is good exercise. What we do not realize is that it brings a richness of practice that will infuse our entire lives. And so the journey of the practice begins as a place for exercise and maybe physical healing. What we find is a wellness that reaches deep to the soul and extends beyond the individual.

Does that mean we all have to practice yoga to be well? From my perspective, I would tell you that we do. But we need to be clear about what yoga is. We have already defined the word 'yoga' as meaning 'to yoke' or 'to integrate.' It is all about being a fully integrated person mentally, physically, and with the world around us. The physical Asanas, or poses, are what we as members of society in the West recognize as yoga. The poses are just one part of the practice that will bring us to a fully integrated state. And really, they can be any kind of movement if we do it with full awareness of the body and mind. We have just scratched the surface of yoga and our potential by beginning to move with awareness.

So where do we start? Take your lead from Patanjali. Begin to practice Ahimsā. Do it first. Just as Patanjali put it down as the first of the Yamas, the first limb in yoga.

If we really want to step onto a path of wellness, the first step is to make the decision to stop harming, or being violent to, ourselves. That is where healing begins and ends leading to wellness like we have not known before. We need to give ourselves permission to take time out, be a little bit 'selfish.' It is okay to tell others no and protect our time. It is okay to get enough sleep and to eat well. And it is definitely okay to find a form of physical exercise that we can personally connect to that brings us a sense of calm and balance.

Make your practice one of exploration. Get to know yourself. What are the things you need to help yourself feel like an integrated person connected to your world? Maybe it is time hiking in the woods, or a massage. Maybe it is just quiet time alone to read a book. Maybe it is taking time for meals and eating better food. Whatever it is, give yourself permission to let go of all your perceived obligations and do something that is just for you. You will be amazed at how quickly all the symptoms of modern life begin to ease and real wellness begins. Now you are beginning to practice Ahmisā at its strongest.

What happens next? As we give ourselves permission to stop harming ourselves, and we start to connect to ourselves as a whole person, we become calmer, less stressed, better rested, and ...

surprise... more able to extend those same feelings around us. Now we have the capacity for the outward practice of non-harming to the world. Start with you, then move on to your family, your friends, your workplace, and the greater society.

You will discover that you suddenly have more time to do the things you have to do as well as the things you have always wanted to do. And you do it with a richness of spirit that feeds everyone around you. And that snowball begins to build. We all will treat each other better. We will find the kindness that so many of us feel is missing. Our society and world will thrive. All because you made a decision to be non-violent.

It is funny how many people actually apologize to me for not practicing yoga. They have all kinds of excuses from not being flexible to how busy their lives are. I used to think that their apologizing to me was so backward. After all, their lack of a yoga practice belonged to them, it had nothing to do with me. As I think about Ahimsā, I realize how wrong I was. While the choice not to practice Western yoga is an individual choice, the real individual practice of yoga – being an integrated person – impacts us all.

Go back to the basics of the *Yoga Sutras*. Come to your Yoga. Through Yoga you will find strength, power, and kindness, like no other. You will be fully well and so will your world.

More information on these
Holistic Coach co-authors
is available at
RadiantCoaches.com.

www.ingramcontent.com/pod-product-compliance
Lightning Source LLC
Chambersburg PA
CBHW021336290326
41933CB00038B/764